Not By Sight

Ministering to Believers Living with Illness and Pain

Wayne and Sherri Connell

Published by WRC2 Media

Copyright © 2004 by Wayne Connell

First Printing 2004
Reprinted 2009, 2014

All Rights Reserved.

For ordering information or special discounts for bulk purchases, contact WRC2 Media P.O. Box 2434 Parker, CO 80134 info@wrc2media.com

Written by Wayne and Sherri Connell
Edited by Carole Mitchell
Cover Design by Wayne Connell

ISBN 978-0-692-20074-2

Not By Sight! is not intended as professional advice. It is solely informational. Please seek the advice of a professional.

A portion of the proceeds support Where Is God Ministries, a 501(c)(3) Non-Profit that ministers to believers living with illness and pain.

Where Is God Ministries
P.O. Box 2345
Parker, Colorado 80134
Website: www.WhereIsGod.net

Contents

About Where Is God Ministries

Often the most difficult part of living with disabling illness or injury is the lack of understanding from others that the person encounters. As healthy, able-bodied people, we might think we have to *see* an outward sign, like a bleeding limb or grey-toned face, before we can *believe* a person is hurting. As a result, when to us they *"look just fine,"* we often disregard what a friend or even a family member is trying to *say*.

Let's face it, most of us cannot comprehend what it is like to be sick or in pain for weeks, months or even years, because we are accustomed to going to the doctor, taking some medication and soon feeling better. Consequently, unless we are educated about what life-changes a chronic condition can cause, we often may inadvertently treat our recently diagnosed loved one as if they need to "snap out of it" or "stop complaining."

Moreover, when the person is a believer, some people often jump to the conclusion that he or she must not "have enough faith" or must be "in sin." Otherwise, why wouldn't God provide healing? Sadly, these assumptions can be exceedingly hurtful and damaging. After all, believers debilitated by illness and pain often live as we all should - *with a dependence on God's strength to carry them through it all.*

To address all these issues, Wayne Connell founded *Where Is God Ministries.* He is joined by pastors and health professionals to reach out to the world with its message of God's strength through suffering. WIGM was designed to help friends and family develop a better understanding of those living with chronic conditions. It also helps us take a deeper look into the Word and acknowledge the extraordinary faith our brothers and sisters have, by God's hand.

WIGM provides articles to help encourage those in their walk with illness and pain, as well as their loved ones to better know how to be a source of encouragement. In addition, WIGM provides helpful links to other sites, resources and organizations.

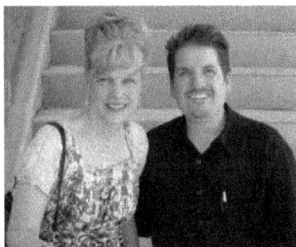

About the Authors

Wayne Connell is the Founder and President of Where Is God Ministries (WIGM). He has a Bachelor's Degree in Liberal Arts from the Colorado Christian University. Wayne founded WIGM as a place of compassion and understanding for believers living with chronic illness and pain. Wayne was inspired to create this organization, because of his wife's battles with illness from a very young age.

Sherri Connell studied Music Theatre for 4 years in college where she was very active in singing and dancing in musicals. She obtained a Bachelor's Degree in Human Resource Management and a Bachelor's degree in Christian Leadership with a minor in Liberal Arts. However, despite plans of a promising career in Human Resource Management and Christian Music ministry, right before beginning her Master's Degree she became very ill with Primary Progressive Multiple Sclerosis and Chronic-Late Lyme Disease. She was then unable to fulfill her lifelong career and theatre dreams.

Although Sherri does not "*look*" disabled to most, for many years she has struggled to wash her hair or go to a doctor's appointment. As a result, she knows first hand the pain and frustration that develops from being trapped inside a body that will no longer cooperate with a person's aspirations or even simple daily chores.

Sherri began writing in her journal to help her cope with the changes in her life. On occasion, she would make copies and pass them out to people to help them understand what she was going through.

One day, Wayne offered to put some of her writing on the internet, so they could ask friends and family to read her thoughts from there. Wayne and Sherri were surprised when they started getting emails from people around the world thanking them for sharing their words and telling stories of how much they had been helped.

Wayne and Sherri quickly recognized the imperative need to educate others on how to be a source of support and encouragement to people with chronic conditions. As a result, Wayne founded, the Invisible Disabilities® Association. It did not take long to realize that believers were grappling with additional concerns, so Wayne also founded, Where Is God Ministries.

Wayne compiled this book with excerpts from Sherri's journal, in order to help other believers communicate their struggles and needs to those around them. Where Is God Ministries distributes this book to give believers living with chronic conditions a voice about how they feel, what they need and how others can be an encouragement! A portion of the proceeds help provide funding for WIGM, a Non-Profit Organization.

Dedication

We would like to dedicate this book to all who live with limitations due to illness and pain. We hope you will find comfort, encouragement and support. Most of all, we pray your loved ones will develop a better understanding of your loss and battles. May their hearts be softened and their eyes opened with compassion, respect and belief for you on your journey.

Acknowledgements and Thanks
From Sherri Connell

I would like to recognize my dear friends and mentors, Dr. Gordon R. Lewis and Dr. Douglas Groothuis. They both have an exemplary expertise of the Bible, achievements in writing and teaching! Both men have encouraged us to follow God's calling for this ministry and have recognized God's hand in taking this mustard seed and growing it into a beautiful tree. They believe in this ministry and the need for the support it gives to so many who are hurting. I praise God for the fellowship with such godly men of wisdom and compassion that I have the privilege to enjoy!

Next, I want to bring my special friend, Sue Bryan, to your attention. At a time when I had given up on finding a friend, she jumped in head-first, right into my life. I was scared and had all of the brick walls built and the security gates closed. Even so, she did not give up, as she kept knocking at my heart's door, until I finally let her in.

Sue, thank you for showing me "God in action." You proved to me God has set up His church, so that we will encourage, love and show compassion to one another. I always felt guilty, because it seemed like being my friend was a burden too hard for anyone to bear. You recognized how much I thoroughly enjoyed helping and doing things for others before the onset of my illness. You reminded me of the joy there was in being available for others *in the midst of my illness* and you encouraged me not to steal that joy from those around me!

You showed me that God has blessings for those who regard their brothers and sisters in times of trouble (Psalm 41:1). Moreover, you pointed out that I and every other child of God has something very valuable to offer. What an eye-opener for me! Not only should I not feel guilty about others helping, but as children of God, we are *called* to help those in need and bear one another's burdens (Galatians 6:2).

You gave me the courage to stand up and say to God's people, "Please listen! Our Lord wants us to love the unlovely and stand by those in times of trouble. We are not to call them *weak* or *blame* them for their conditions. We are not to act like we have all of the answers. Instead, we are to come *along side* of them, whether they are in the pit of a volcano or on top of a beautiful mountain!" For the Bible calls us to *weep* with our brothers and sisters as well as *rejoice* with them (Romans 12:15 & 16).

Finally, I cannot possibly make a list of names of all who have helped me now and then with groceries and rides to doctor appointments, but I don't want to fail to recognize my friend Nancy Ballard. She has not only given up countless hours of her time to drive me to various appointments, but has been a *real friend*, by allowing me to be honest and unlovely at times...Okay, many times!

Foreword
Seeing Invisible Disabilities

Jesus had an uncanny way of seeing what others missed and ministering to those who were forgotten, shunned, or misunderstood. He touched and healed the lepers when everyone else scurried away. He cared for those with chronic afflictions--such as congenital blindness and incurable hemorrhage--while others gave up. He bestowed hope where others scattered the ashes of despair. He was love Incarnate (John 1:14; 1 John 4:16). We need that character of divine love if we are to see and minister to the hurts of others.

America has made some strides in recognizing and assisting people with disabilities. Most public facilities are now accessible to the handicapped. The pool where I swim has a lift for the disabled. The law rightly forbids discriminating against the handicapped (see Leviticus 19:14, Deuteronomy 27:18, Matthew 25:40). In the Christian community, Joni Eareckson Tada has raised people's awareness of the needs of those who suffer from severe disabilities. She has encouraged the afflicted not to despair but to trust God to use their broken lives for the glory of God and the good of others.

Despite these gains in awareness, many disabled people continue to suffer in two ways: from their chronic physical distress and from misunderstanding. Their suffering is masked by a healthy appearance. They are not in wheelchairs and do not use canes. Yet their pain and debility is real and chronic. They have "invisible disabilities." It may be the soul-sapping fatigue, environmental sensitivity, and chronic pain of fibromyalgia, or lupus, or Lyme disease, or multiple sclerosis.

These souls suffer not only from their diseases but often from the uninformed and hurtful reactions of others.

Those suffering from fibromyalgia, such as my wife, often ricochet from one physician to another, repeatedly encountering the impatience and defeatism that often characterize the medical community's attitude toward those who suffer from ailments that are intractable, invisible and (usually) non-terminal. Insurance routinely refuses to cover needed treatments for these conditions. Worse yet, their loved ones frequently do not understand the nature of their invisible disability and respond wrongly. When someone looks healthy, we are tempted to tell them to "buck up" and do what we think they should do. Those with invisible disabilities are often expected to do what is beyond them. We would never tell someone who uses a cane to run a marathon, but going to the store may be a marathon for someone with lupus. A seminary student of mine looks healthy, yet he suffers from such chronic and extreme back pain that it caused him to lose his medical practice. He also lost a friend who could not accept the limitations that chronic illness put on their relationship.

What can Christians do to discern invisible disabilities and display the love of Christ? First, we can empathize with them, instead of lecturing or ignoring them. The Letter of Hebrews tells us to remember those in prison as though we were shackled with them (Hebrews 13:3). Similarly, we must try to put ourselves into the prison of the chronically ill person's life. This is difficult, and almost nothing in our hedonistic popular culture encourages it. Nevertheless, we need empathy to be agents of love and encouragement. Jesus wept; so must we (John 11:35). Second, we should listen to and believe what the afflicted tell us. My wife looks so healthy and fit that someone in the locker room where we swim thought she was another woman who had been swimming at top speed for an hour straight. But if you truly listen to Rebecca's story--a story of pain and frustration mixed with faith and determination--you will find that things are quite different from how they appear. Third, Wayne and Sherri Connell's web site, The Invisible Disabilities Association (www.InvisibleDisabilities.org) offers a wealth of materials, including the book, *But You LOOK Good*. Sherri, who suffers from an invisible disability, has a big heart, an indomitable spirit, and much practical and spiritual advice concerning these heartbreaking problems.

Let us seek to have the eyes of Jesus, so we may look beyond appearances and gaze deeply into the lives of those who are suffering. Then we can offer them our love, understanding, and encouragement.

- Douglas Groothuis, Ph.D.

Dr. Groothuis is a professor at The Denver Seminary in Colorado. He is the author of Truth Decay, On Jesus, On Pascal and many more. He is also the husband of Rebecca Merrill Groothuis, a writer and editor. Visit Doug and Rebecca's website at: www.DougGroothuis.com.

Part One

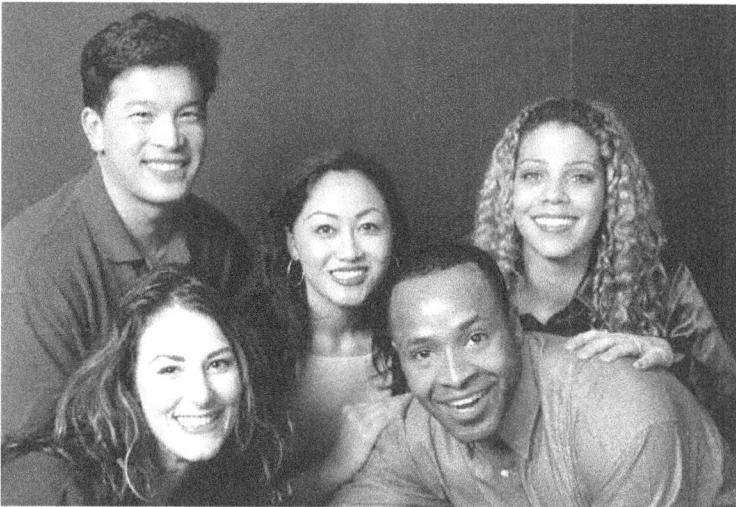

Ministering to Believers Living with Illness and Pain

The King will answer and say to them,
"Truly I say to you, to the extent that you
Did it to one of these brothers of Mine,
Even the least of them, you did it to Me."

Matthew 25:40 NASB

Chapter One
The Heartbreak of Seeing Them Suffer

Witnessing a loved one battle a debilitating condition can be stressful, baffling and painful! It "...often makes people feel helpless and uncomfortable, and they may behave in awkward ways or simply feel the need to create distance. Their emotions of fear, disappointment, and loss are often complicated by feelings of guilt for being healthy or for having needs that [they] may not be able to meet"[1] explained Lisa Lorden, a writer who lives with Fibromyalgia.

As loving friends and family members, we hate to see our loved ones hurting, but we really do not know how to help or what to say. Pauline Boss, PhD a professor of Family Social Science at The University of Minnesota revealed, "...the ambiguity surrounding the illness keeps people confused, so they don't know what to do or what decisions to make."[2] When we think of something we are sure will help, we are often met with an irritated reaction from our suffering friend or family member. This response makes us wonder where he or she is coming from and why our loved one is so sensitive.

Regrettably, people can easily fall prey to disbelieving their loved ones, because they appear to "look" fine, even though they say they are not. It is difficult for those who are healthy to understand this perplexity. Sometimes it is easier to come to the conclusion that they are exaggerating the extent of their situation or even making it up. 'Peoples' observations do not conform to their expectation as to what a sick person should look and act like," examined Lisa Copen, the founder of Rest Ministries. "Therefore they are quick to become intolerant and suspect that the symptoms are overstated."[3]

Despite the fact that we expect our loved ones to "look sick," as we did when we were in bed with the flu, they usually do not. Why? Well, because they don't have the flu. Their condition does not always produce the symptoms that make them look so flush and drawn. While most people in severe pain wince and moan until the pain subsides, someone in chronic pain makes great efforts to walk upright, smile and enjoy life. For them, they can no longer wait for the pain to leave - *they must try to move on.*

The truth is even though we assume someone with an ongoing condition is going to look sick or in pain, "Many with chronic physical illness look no different than other people, so family members and friends may not realize why they are preoccupied with pain or their prognosis"[4] Thus, we must learn to *listen* and *believe* our loved ones when they tell us of their struggles, whether we can "see" it or not.

What is more, when people live with a debilitating condition, they often lose the ability to participate in various degrees of activities they have always enjoyed. Some only contend with minor adjustments and are still able to lead full active lives. Some learn to set boundaries and modify tasks and activities to avoid flare-ups. Others, tragically, lose careers, hobbies and struggle to get through daily living.

Douglas Groothuis, PhD, an author and husband of a writer and editor living with Fibromyalgia shared, "A seminary student of mine looks healthy, yet he suffers from such chronic and extreme back pain that he lost his medical practice. He also lost a friend who could not accept the limitations that chronic illness put on their relationship."[5]

These losses are very real and can be devastating. Still, we often do not think of the inability to participate in an activity as a *loss*, as in the death of a loved one. Therefore, we often fail to advance through the proper stages of grief and loss *with* our loved one. Instead of addressing the situation so that we can adapt and cope alongside our suffering friend or family member, we often choose to remain in denial. Boss described those who are in relationship to a chronically ill person as "Cognitively immobilized, many choose irrational responses; they close out the ill person, and act as if he or she is already dead and gone. Or they deny the illness exists, and interact with the ill person as if nothing were wrong."[6]

We may even claim our loved one is failing to follow the doctor's advice or is not trying hard enough. We often assume that modern medicine must have something to get the patient back to normal functioning. But, treating chronic conditions is not always that simple: "Chronic illness rarely responds to a direct intervention, and by definitions, is elusive of cure,"[7] admitted F. Marcus Brown III, PhD, a therapist who specializes in chronic illness. Therefore, we cannot jump to the conclusion our suffering loved ones are sick because they have failed *to try* to get well.

Often we tell our loved ones they need to "look at the bright side" or "have a positive attitude." We do not take into account the loss and struggles they encounter on a regular basis and we seem to disregard the incredible attitude they have already displayed.

"The individual living with chronic illness has a history of health, has felt well and lively, and has independently pursued goals and dreams" declared Jackson P. Rainer, Ph.D, a leading authority on grief and loss. "As the illness progresses, she must adjust each day to the disease, sometimes severe, sometimes in remission, and always present. The sense of health and vibrancy is, at best, diminished, and at worst, lost."[8]

Other times, we begin to question why God would allow them to suffer. We know our Lord is fair and just, so we may tragically assume that it must be the fault of our loved one. "We tend to take health, family, food, and other blessings as being our birthright. The thought does not come easily that these are blessings that we don't deserve, that God is free to either give or withhold"[9] explained Jeffrey Boyd, MD, a psychiatrist who writes and lectures on coping with chronic conditions.

We might even jump to the conclusion that our loved ones must lack enough faith to be healed or they are caught up in a secret sin. Therefore, we bombard them with books, tapes and even Scripture in effort to convince them that if they followed all the proper steps, they would no longer be ill.

This is not how God intends for us to come along side our brother or sister. There are no fancy words or formulas to make God give us what we want. He is not a genie we can take out of the bottle to perform our every wish. We may continue to ask Him for healing and have complete faith that He can, but only if it is His will.

All the same, we must learn how to be sensitive to our friend or family member. We cannot treat this dear person as if he or she is at fault, lack faith or are not trying hard enough to get better. It is one thing to share information as a gesture of support and quite another to attack our loved one's most valuable sustenance – *her faith and relationship with the Lord.*

The purpose of this book is to shed a light on ongoing illness and pain. In Part Two, we will discuss some of our natural responses to someone debilitated by illness or pain and why our kind efforts may not be helpful. We will also address some reactions we, as believers, are tempted to give and why they can be hurtful.

Some of these examples may seem perfectly appropriate to us, while others may be obviously unacceptable. Either way, this book will help us all to see why our *well-meaning* comments may not be *well-received.* In Part Three, by mapping out some steps of how to be a source of encouragement, we will learn how to positively respond to our loved one's illness and needs, what to say and why.

Our hope in making this book available is to bring friends, family members and loved ones together to a compassionate understanding, by untangling the perplexities of how to be a true foundation of support. Moreover, we endeavor to make evident what unsung heroes those living with chronic conditions are, so that we may all see the battle they are fighting with *courage, perseverance* and most of all… *faith.*

Part Two

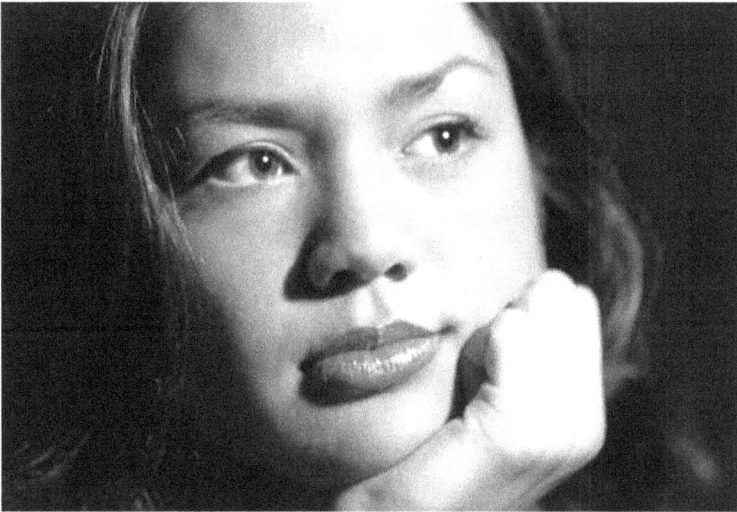

Recognizing Our
Discouraging Responses

Before destruction the heart of man is haughty,
But humility goes before honor.
He who gives an answer before he hears,
It is folly and shame to him.

Proverbs 18: 12 & 13 NASB

Chapter Two
Struggling With What to Say

Have you ever felt frustrated, because you never seem to know how to show that you care? When you think you have the perfect thing to say, does your loved one get upset with you? Here you are, being supportive and trying to help, but they look at you as if you said something horrible!

Cathy, a woman who lives with Multiple Sclerosis wrote, "Usually family members and loved ones do not intentionally try to cause us harm - they think they're being helpful. When in fact, they are not helpful and cause us emotional hardships and undue anxieties."[1]

We truly care about our loved ones and hate to see them hurting! We want so desperately to "make it all go away" or to at least minimize its affects. However, in our attempts to "make it all better," we sometimes seem to make it worse. It does not make any sense to us, because in our minds we are really helping and coming up with some great solutions.

As believers, we often grapple even deeper with the pain of seeing someone dealing with loss and difficulty! It breaks our heart knowing our loved one is struggling, so we search for answers, hope and promise that we can find a formula to make it end. Nevertheless, when we share our advice, we are not always met with gratitude. We do not understand why, because to us we are sharing God's promises and giving wonderful suggestions.

We must ask ourselves how we treat someone who claims to be

sick or in pain, even though he or she may look fine to us. Are we understanding, when he tells us he is unable to work or help with ministries? What do we do when we cannot deal with the enormity of the situation? How do we react to the person who says she is still suffering from something we think should have been long gone by now? Do we fear the prospect of suffering so much that we insist God does not allow it?

In the following four chapters, we will address some of our common responses and discuss several of our reactions based on these responses. We will also give samples of comments we may make and explain why these approaches can be discouraging.

Chapter Three
But They LOOK So Good

Since They LOOK Good, They Must FEEL Good

But, you don't LOOK sick! But, you LOOK fine to me!
But, you are here, so you must be feeling well!
But, you LOOK like you are doing great!

"To a healthy person, none of these comments seem unusual or insincere. Our friends are simply trying to find the right thing to say."[1] But to the person receiving the remark, it can be quite aggravating. Charlene, a woman with Graves Disease and Fibromyalgia agreed, "I was just telling a friend this morning if one more person says you don't look sick, or you look fine I was going to scream!"[2]

One of the biggest complaints people debilitated by illness or pain have, is that others do not believe what they say because they "LOOK good" to everyone else. The bottom line is that "Peoples' observations do not conform to their expectation as to what a sick person should look and act like." Copen illustrated. "Therefore they are quick to become intolerant and suspect that the symptoms are overstated."[3]

When we think of someone who is sick, we think of a person who is in bed looking flushed, with messed up hair. After all, most of us look pretty bad when we are down with a virus. Furthermore, when someone tells us they are in pain, we expect to see them wincing. "Although people do sympathize with pain, it is under circumstances that we believe are severely painful, such as childbirth, trauma, late stages of cancer, etc." Copen illustrated. "People cannot relate with the chronically ill since the individual is not screaming, crying or grimacing."[4]

On the contrary, most people with chronic conditions look very normal. Debbie, another woman with MS added, "I have MS and I can not make my husband understand he can not *see* how I feel."[5] First, chronically ill people do not always have the fever that causes the washed out look. Second, when a person is in pain much of the time, she eventually learns to put on the make-up or a smile and try to enjoy life as much as possible.

Because of this, we sometimes assume that when our loved ones are looking good, smiling and laughing they must be "feeling good." Bek Oberin, a lady who writes on living with Chronic Fatigue Syndrome appealed, "Please understand the difference between 'happy' and 'healthy.' When you've got the flu you probably feel miserable with it, but I've been sick for years. I can't be miserable all the time, in fact I work hard at *not* being miserable."[6] This is the idea of having a truly positive attitude: *feeling* a sense of misery but working hard and not *succumbing* to complete misery.

Of course, our loved ones are grateful when they do not look sick! Yet, it jabs like a knife when others say it in a way in which they are really implying, "I don't believe what you are telling me, because I cannot see it for myself" or "Well, it must not be that bad, because you look fine." Pat, a woman with Fibromyalgia wrote, "I want to get a t-shirt and a sweat shirt printed with, 'I feel worse than I look.' That way, maybe people wouldn't always be telling me how good I look, when inside I feel like I've been hit by a Mack truck."[7]

They Must Be Fine, Because They are Out and About

You made it, so you must be feeling good today!
You are here, so you must be doing well!
I know you are okay, when you are here.

When we see someone, whom we know has been struggling, out and about, we can get so excited for him or her! After all, this must mean they are feeling good, right? Well, not exactly. It is easy to jump to this conclusion, because when most people are really sick, they usually do not get out until they are feeling better. But for those who do not have enough good days to get things done, they do not have the luxury of waiting for a good day in order to run errands and live life.

Those who are debilitated by their conditions need to get out and enjoy people once in a while, too. They want to laugh, talk and look their best, like everyone else, but this can seem confusing to onlookers. Lorden expounded, "Around others, it's difficult to know how to act because we're caught between contradictory wishes: wanting to appear normal and wanting to be understood. So what can we do?"[8]

Sometimes the chronically ill are so sick they *should* be in bed, but they push themselves to go to church or a function, because they need the spiritual food and fellowship – not because they are suddenly feeling well. "Of course, [people] really do believe that you must be feeling better or you wouldn't be out of bed" Copen admitted. "Those of us, who are ill, however, understand that if we stayed in bed until we felt better, we would never leave the bedroom and we would miss out on life. So we get out of bed."[9]

No matter how great they may appear, we cannot comprehend what it took for them to get ready, how much pain they endured while they were there and how much worse they will be for days or even weeks from the endeavor.

They Should Stop Asking for Help and Start Helping

Why don't you try reaching out to others?
It will make you feel better.
Why don't you get involved in a ministry, so you are not so focused on yourself?

Asking a person to get more involved may be a great idea for someone who is able to care for his or her basic needs and is still functioning with little limitation. After all, there are people with all types of dysfunctions and disabilities that are mild enough to still be able to work or volunteer. Or, it might be a feasible suggestion for someone whose symptoms are fairly controlled, therefore allowing them to have many good days. It may even be reasonable for someone who has moderate symptoms, but is still able to do a little bit above their daily activities.

We must be sensitive to those who are struggling to get through a day at work and have great difficulty doing much else. For them, it is all they can do to get dinner or pick up a few things around the house. Many are no longer able to work at a job, but "work" all day to meet daily needs like showering, making meals and shopping. Their day is like climbing a mountain, trying to get a few things done around the house, making appointments and filling out medical paperwork. They may even be spending all of their time and energy getting tests, treatments and surgeries.

In all, why would we expect a person who is in a position of requiring assistance themselves in order to get their daily needs met, to be able to help others? Let us listen carefully to our brothers and sisters. Most likely, they are mourning not being able to help, as they would love to be able. We might make them feel worse about it than they already do. Maybe if we offer to help with their groceries, meals or rides to appointments, they could use their energy to be part of a ministry again!

They Should Get a Job

The Bible says if you don't work, you're not entitled to food and shelter.
You could at least work part-time!
You don't look disabled!

Healthy people often have a difficult time understanding why a person who looks fine may not be able to work. It is tragic, but some of us react as much as to claim the person does not want to work. Some well meaning people even take Scripture out of context to prove that everyone, even a disabled person, is required to work. Yes, there are many lazy people in this world. But it is devastating when someone who has a legitimate illness or injury is accused of choosing not to do what they would love to be able to do, like working.

If people with disabilities, whether the disabilities are visible to us or not, are wrongly accused of being lazy or unwilling to "cheer up," false witness is being borne against them (Ex 20:16). Those who are healthy need to be mindful not to place blame and false accusations on those who live with persistent illness, pain or disability.

It is a travesty when an honest, ethical person who has lost much of their independence and dreams is treated as if they are trying to get out of life's responsibilities. Many accuse them of trying to get attention and a free ride. Contrary to popular belief, people living with chronic conditions do not receive a lot of notice and fan-fare in the long-run. In reality, many lose their careers, their friends, their family members and even their spouses. Truth be known, they are often avoided, isolated, lonely and without the help that they need.

They CHOOSE Not to Be Involved

You're lucky you don't have to help out on Sundays!
You should get more involved, it would make you feel better!

Even in church, there can be resentment towards people with debilitating illness, because they are not able to help as much as they would like to or even at all. It is very difficult to understand how they can say they are unable to lend a hand, when they look perfectly capable.

Here is something we have to ask ourselves: What if, for example, a person living with Lupus were asked to help with the nursery on Sundays, but said "no?" Would we think they were giving an excuse, because to us they look perfectly able? After all, if we see them in church smiling and talking, doesn't that show they are doing fine? Doesn't it mean they can function like that all of the time? If they can show up for church, why can't they work in the nursery or help elsewhere?

The fact is, even though they *look* fine for one hour a week, does not mean chronically ill people *feel* fine and it does not mean they would be able to do more than attend. The heartbreaking truth is they would *love* to be able to help with the children or be more involved. It tears them up inside to not be able to be an active part of church ministry!

As healthy people, we do not always think about the huge mountain they had to climb to get to church on Sunday morning. Then, sitting and listening during the service and visiting afterwards can be a tremendous endeavor. What's more, we do not see the costly price in the days following they end up paying from pushing themselves so hard to make it. No, to expect them to do more than they can, when getting to church is such a struggle, would be ludicrous.

Chapter Four
What's The Big Deal?

It Can't Be THAT Bad

Hey, it could be worse! At least you are not bedridden!
Yes, but you LOOK good! Oh, you'll be alright!

Dealing with illness/injury is a challenge that can be heartbreaking and scary. Because we love them, the last thing we want to do is to see them hurting. When our loved ones are first diagnosed, we rally around them and do whatever we can to help them! When they do not improve, we feel helpless. We know we cannot make it all go away, so we at least try to ease the magnitude of what is happening to them. We think that if we can make them see that what they are going through is not so terrible, maybe they could deal with it better.

This response allows us to better cope with the issue ourselves and we think it will allow our loved ones to do the same. On the other hand, it may make our loved ones think we have no clue what they are going through, because we keep down-playing, or minimizing it. Besides, we cannot show compassion, empathy and support if we are telling them, "it is no big deal." Linda, a woman living with MS expressed her frustration when she questioned, "Why can't people understand I don't have a cold. I have MS!"[1]

If we cannot acknowledge that what our loved ones are going through is *real* and as difficult as they are experiencing, then how can we show kindness? We cannot be compassionate about a situation if we are telling ourselves the situation does not even exist! What's more, how sensitive is it to refuse to meet them where they are and where they are hurting, only to blurt out, "It could be worse!"

I Know, I Can Relate

I know what you mean. Ya, I am tired all the time, too."
Join the club. Ya, I need someone to clean my house, too!

It is natural to try to show someone we can relate in a difficult situation. Most of us find ourselves doing it all the time! If we try to prove we can relate to their suffering or situation, then we are expressing our ability to comprehend the issue and we are displaying our capability to understand. Nonetheless, it can backfire if a healthy person tries to claim they know what it is like to have a chronic illness, because they get "tired" too or because they need help getting things done as well.

People in good health may get *tired* after they have been shopping, car-pooling, working, volunteering, cleaning, cooking and running around. People with unremitting conditions, however, often feel horrible, unbelievably exhausted, dizzy, nauseas and/or are in severe pain with or without even doing much or anything at all to bring it on. Julie, with Multiple Sclerosis showed her aggravation over people thinking they know what it is like to have MS, when she noted, "I just hate it when people say, 'Oh, I'm always forgetting things too' or 'I'm tired as well... so much to do.' I'm tired of trying to explain it's completely different."[2]

The truth is, even though overall healthy people may know what it is like to be "worn out" from a busy day, they cannot have any idea of what it is like to have bone-crushing fatigue and immobilizing pain from an illness or injury unless they have suffered the same themselves. They may even know what it is like have more things "to do" than they can get done, but they will never know the constant frustrations of not being able to achieve anywhere near the magnitude of activities a healthy person can accomplish. Nor can they comprehend what it is like to struggle to do a few things that everyone else is taking for granted. Furthermore, while most are complaining they cannot get *everything* done, those with disabilities may be trying to get *something* done.

It Must Be Nice

It must be great to always be on vacation.
What do you do all day, lie around and watch TV?
It must be nice not to have to work!

Around those who are suffering, disabled or chronically ill, we often feel uncomfortable with the situation, so we try to lighten up the seriousness by joking about how easy they have it. We kid about how wonderful it would be to lie around all day and not have to work. What we do not realize is that they hate having to rest and would rather be active. Instead of showing our compassion, we tell them they are lucky to be sick! Can you imagine losing some or many of the things you loved most in life and being told that you are *lucky?*

Additionally, we often complain about being "busy" as if those with disabilities sit around at home with nothing to do. Yet, do we get more done on our list when we are healthy or when we are sick? For most, the chores pile up even more when they are ill, but typically healthy people can get their list of chores done in a day or two when their illness passes. As a result, it is illogical to think that people who have conditions that are debilitating are lying around with nothing to do! If they are lying down, it is because they *have* to, not because they *want* to.

Besides, while most healthy people are busy living life to the fullest, those debilitated by illness and injury are booked up with making doctor appointments, sitting in waiting rooms, seeing doctors, filling out paperwork, getting prescriptions, getting tests done, having procedures, taking their medications and trying to get through the day.

People in good health may think it is a hassle to work, run errands, clean the house, work on the yard, travel, shop and cook. In contrast, those who have been unable to do these things, yearn for the day they could achieve so much! They grieve for the loss of being able to do "ordinary" tasks and consider them a blessing, not a chore. It is hard to fathom that some people can even begin to think that a person is better off being sick or in pain and spending hours upon hours dealing with their medical condition, than able to work or actively enjoy life!

They Are Just Complainers

Everyone has their cross to bear.
You should count your blessings. Be positive.
God helps those who help themselves."

Yes, we all have our cross to bear. Somehow we think that if someone has an illness, that is his or her cross while ours is something else like dealing with a difficult childhood. What we do not realize is that those suffering often deal with all of the same things we do in addition to their disability. They have marriage problems and financial difficulties like the next person. They can even have additional pressures of loss of income, increased medical bills, lack of ability to care for the home and added stress to the spouse and children. Moreover, they must deal with life's complications while they are sick, spending much of their time at the doctors' office and filling out endless paperwork.

It is so easy to assume that when a person is discussing their situation, they are failing to count their blessings. The irony is, when someone is limited by symptoms that causes them to give up many activities in their lives, they actually *do* count their blessings. In fact, they often give thanks for being able to do something about which most people do not even think twice! Thus, they give thanks when they are able to do the smallest of things that most people never even blink an eye at.

Think about it. When was the last time you took the time to thank God for being able to sleep for six hours straight or for giving you the strength to wash your hair? Have you ever praised Him for being able to scrub your toilet or refilling your soap dispensers? Do you rejoice after making it to and from the grocery store without collapsing? Have you ever given thanks for being able to dust a few pieces of furniture or making a simple meal?

No, people who have disabilities count blessings others rarely stop to think about! They even count the wonderful things in life everyone else is taking for granted and calling a "chore." Dreaded tasks for most are dreams realized for them. Subsequently, when they can do them, they count them! Wow! What a positive attitude it takes to count such blessings that others do not even give a thought and even loathe! Even if they did complain…so what? Most people complain after being sick or in pain after a day or so! What courage to endure it for a lifetime!

They Expect Too Much From Others

He doesn't want to work and expects everyone else to do it for him!
She wants the church to do everything for her!
She whines and wants a free ride!

Many times we fear that people who have disabilities are going to expect us to fill their every demand. For people whose disabilities are not so obvious (or invisible), we may even suspect that they are being "needy." So, we often avoid those people who we think are trying to get attention and are expecting the church to do everything for him or her.

Besides, our members are already involved in so many ministries, we do not have abundant time to make countless visits to a person's home and run their errands. Sometimes we realize the need is real, but fear it is too overwhelming. On the contrary, there are many ways to help someone with physical obstacles that really do not take much time. To a person with limitations, even the smallest gesture can mean so much and be a tremendous help!

Chapter Five

I Can't Handle It

I Won't Accept It

It's all in your head! You'll feel better soon!
Oh, you're fine! Don't worry about it.

When we are faced with any type of tragic situation, our most natural instinct is to go into denial. This reaction is built inside of us, so we can have time to let it sink in and not go into shock. Next, we should move into acceptance, grief and coping. However, many people often remain in denial when the illness continues, because we do not want to think about the losses and changes.

We might think this is the most helpful reaction, but it is actually the most hurtful for everyone. By refusing to acknowledge what our loved ones are going through, we fail to allow them, *and ourselves,* to advance through the proper steps of grief and loss. This is the healthiest way to process the changes and learn to cope with the future. Pastor Rick Warren clarified, "Whenever we try to avoid or escape the difficulties of life, we short-circuit the process, delay our growth, and actually end up with a worse kind of pain – the worthless type that accompanies denial and avoidance."[1] Additionally, our friend or family member is left to mourn their losses and make adjustments alone.

Even though we are afraid that recognizing the illness means accepting its fate, nothing could be further from the truth. "What? Accept the illness?" asked author Kathleen Lewis. "Most people choose to see the acceptance of a chronic illness as either complete capitulation or total vigilance. In reality, it is neither. Acceptance of an illness can be an integral part of getting on with life."[2]

When we acknowledge the existence of the illness, we are simply taking into consideration there is a hurdle to jump over. If we do not admit that the hurdle is even there, how can we plan our crusade to get over it? Doesn't it make more sense to declare there is a war to be fought, so we can make a battle plan, rather than ignoring the war and hoping it will go away?

I Want Them To Be Better

Feeling good today? Doing good this week?
Having a good day? You better yet?
But, you sound like you are doing really well!

Instead of asking our loved ones, "How are they feeling?" we often try to put words in their mouth by asking, "Feeling good today?" or "Having a good day?" By stating our questions like this, we are telling them what we want to hear and we are not giving them the opportunity to answer with the truth. We do this, because we want to hear that answer. We love them and are hoping against hope they are better!

All the same, this can be frustrating when we try to force them to say they are feeling well, when they are not. This puts them into the position of either having to be dishonest to make us happy or to tell the truth and sound negative. "This seemingly innocuous ritual of polite conversation is fraught with complexity and emotion for me." Lorden shared. "I wish I could be like other people who can reply,

'Fine thanks' without a second thought. But when discouraging and painful symptoms are overwhelming, this simple response feels like a lie."[3]

Sometimes we may even call someone on the phone we have not spoken with in a while. Low and behold, they sound great! They seem chipper, energetic and really good! What we do not realize is that they may simply be elated to be getting our call! They may be happy and surprised or relieved because we ended their isolation! Maybe they are trying to be joyful, despite their circumstance. Likewise, they know that if they sound gloomy and miserable every time we call, that we may never call again.

We often jump to the conclusion they are better and say, "Wow! You must be feeling great today!" Unfortunately, we do not listen when they tell us they are not. We start insisting, "Oh, come on! I can tell you are better! I can hear it!" That can be extremely difficult for our loved ones, because they were simply trying to be positive, now we are suddenly accusing them of not being honest with us. When we want to know if they are better, we should ask them; but we must be willing to hear the *truth*.

For those whose symptoms do not remit and are constant, we should not expect them to suddenly feel great. If they do, I am sure they will tell us! For those who do have conditions that go into remission or flare on occasion, they do enjoy telling others about their good days. Overall, when we want to know how they are feeling, we should ask! If we do not really want to know the truth, we should *not* ask!

They Should Push Harder

Oh, you could do it if you wanted to.
If you can do that, why can't you do this?
You would feel better if you got out more.

It is perfectly normal and easy to forget about our loved ones' illnesses! When people are standing there looking like they are fine, we often forget about their limitations. Because of this, we sometimes treat them as if they are using their illness as an excuse or trying to pull the wool over our eyes when they say they are unable to do something. In this case, we must respect their answer and realize it does not mean they do not *want* to, it means they *can't*.

Sometimes we question how they can do one thing, but not another. "Please understand that being able to stand up for five minutes doesn't necessarily mean that I can stand up for ten minutes, or an hour." Oberin appealed. "It's quite likely that doing that five minutes has exhausted my resources and I'll need to recover - imagine an athlete after a race. They couldn't repeat that feat right away either."[4]

We even question how they seemed able to do something one day, but now they say they cannot. "It's quite possible…that one day I am able to walk to the park and back, while the next day I'll have trouble getting to the kitchen" Oberin continued. "Please don't attack me when I'm ill by saying, 'But you did it before!' If you want me to do something, ask if I can and I'll tell you."[5]

Often we have difficulty understanding how something that seems so easy and enjoyable to us, can be too strenuous for them. Even so, they know how painful something will be, how much their condition will worsen and how much of a negative affect it will have on them afterwards. "Please understand that 'getting out and doing things' does not make me feel better, and can often make me seriously worse" Oberin pled. "Telling me that I need some fresh air and exercise is not appreciated and not correct - if I could do it, I would."[6] Thus, even if we think it might do them some good; this is something only *they* can decide. After all, if it *did* make them feel better to get out, don't we think that they would be getting out all the time?

There's Got To Be An Answer

Couldn't you work part-time or work from home?
Can't you take some pain medication?
This too shall pass.

We have all done it! We come across someone with a problem, so we come up with an idea. We hate to see them hurting, so if we can fix it then we all win! Yet, sometimes we want so badly for our suggestions to work, that we fail to listen to the person with the illness. He may try to tell us he has attempted this treatment already or that he is not a candidate for the medication.

Despite the facts, we keep on insisting we have the answer. Other times, our ideas are preposterous and only make her realize we have no idea what she is going through. For example, if a person can no longer work at their desk job, why would we recommend she take in some laundry to make some money? If she is struggling to take a shower and get her meals each day, why would we advise her to work a part-time job?

We even try to fix our loved one with quick Scripture or proverbial sayings. True, sharing Scripture is what we all should do! When a fellow brother or sister is in need, God's Word is our bread of life. It can bring us comfort, strength and growth. Spending time reading the Bible and talking with God gives hope, joy and peace in the midst of the storm (Phil 4:7).

Nevertheless, let us not flippantly toss out passages for the purpose of shrugging off the situation and downplaying its impact on their lives. "Avoid giving 'God balm,' If you say 'God will heal you' or 'all things work together...' she will believe you don't really understand and avoid sharing her feelings with you in the future."[7]

Let us share Scripture and be in the Word together. But let us not watch our friend freeze out in the storm, while we sit idly by the fire shouting, "Don't worry! This too shall pass!" Instead, we should go out into the cold to offer our brother a coat. We may get wet and we may even get a chill, but we will soon dry out. There is certainly no quick fix and may be no words of true comfort. But a warm embrace to a friend in pain will mean everything to them.

God Must Heal Them

God cannot use a broken body.
God promised to heal you." Why won't you let Him?
It's God's Will for you to be healed.

It is very important to pray for healing with those who are ill or in pain. Oftentimes people are released of their spiritual and physical bondages of the past, un-forgiveness, sin and oppression. Those are all issues that must be addressed, because they can cause very real physical and emotional symptoms.

However, when we continue to insist on healing by barraging our loved ones with Scripture taken out of context and offer to take them to a "healer," they can feel quite spiritually beat up. "My friend is always trying to get me to go to a healing service with her" Lewis recalled a lady once told her. "She will call and ask me how I feel and then proceed to quote me scriptures and end up acting like I'm really not as bad as I feel."[8]

Honestly, we all want to see our loved ones healed of their condition. There is nothing wrong with praying for healing! In fact, we should continue to take our petitions to the Lord (Eph 6:18). Then again, we often go down the list to find out what they are doing wrong that is keeping God from healing them. This can cause great frustration, resentment, guilt and disappointment for our loved one to be blamed for not being healed. Many even become afraid to go to church, because of the accusations. How devastating that is, right down to the core of the Holy Spirit that lives within us.

The Bible is very clear that this earth is full of sin, disease and trials (Rom 8:18-22). This world is fallen and imperfect and we, as Christians are neither immune to illness nor live in a bubble of protection from tribulation. A well-known author, Max Lucado said, "We're not supposed to feel at home here. In fact, pain on earth is God's reminder that we're not made for this world."[9]

What many of us, even as believers, do not want to accept is that God does not always *choose* to heal everyone in the way *we* think is best. Instead, sometimes our Lord chooses to allow His children to have a thorn in their flesh (2 Cor 12:7). The apostle Paul was not healed of his thorn, though he prayed earnestly and faithfully (2 Cor 12:8 & 9). Despite Paul's divine ability to heal others (Acts 28:9), later he apparently could not heal either Epaphroditus (Phil 2:25) or Trophimus (2 Tim 4:20).

When we feel like demanding God to remove our suffering, we must ask ourselves, "Why would God exempt us from what he allowed his own Son to experience?"[10] Paul himself concluded, "I consider that our present sufferings are not worth comparing with the glory that will be revealed in us" (Rom 8:18). After all, "…we share in his sufferings in order that we may also share in his glory" (Rom 8:17b).

"Jesus Christ is the Great Physician and He has all authority and power to work miracles, but He does not always answer our prayers in the way we may think best…. wholeness is not dependent upon circumstances or the condition of our physical or emotional being" expounded free-lance writer, singer and speaker, Laurie Thompson. "Wholeness only comes from within--from a relationship with Jesus Christ! My body may seem 'broken' to some people, but I am just as whole as any other person."[11]

Chapter Six

They Must Be Doing Something Wrong

They're Not TRYING To Get Better

Maybe you should push yourself more.
Aren't you taking anything for it?
I thought there was a cure for that!

It is so easy when we are feeling healthy to assume that we are, because we are doing all of the right things. We take our vitamins to keep us well and we take our medicine when we are not. Subsequently, wouldn't it be logical to conclude that people continue to be sick, because they are not taking care of themselves or doing what their doctor is telling them to do?

Maybe they have failed to try hard enough to find the right doctor who has all of the answers. After all, if they were doing what they were supposed to be doing, they would recover. The sad truth is that *"You're still sick?"* is a question [people with chronic illness] commonly have to field even after 10 or 20 years of illness. Joan S. Livingston, an author who lives with CFIDS exclaimed. "The implication—a punch to the gut—is that you're not really trying or just haven't scouted out the right doctor."[1]

If people are in pain, we often assume they must not be taking pain medication. Since 2000, I have been battling with constant, unbearable, shooting, nerve pain that causes spasms, seizures and severe sleep deprivation. This pain is the most mind-boggling, unbelievable pain I have ever experienced and it feels like being tortured with razors and acid.

My journal entries remind me of thoughts I've had over the years that it amazes me how many people have asked me if I had tried ibuprofen, aspirin or sleeping pills! Of course I have tried those as well as dozens of prescription drugs, pain ointments, patches, supplements, therapies and surgeries. Boy, do I feel like people think I must really be dense when they ask if I have tried an over the counter pain reliever. Do they really think I have been going without sleep for several years, without even trying something?

Managing ongoing pain and symptoms is not always as easy as popping a few pills to make it disappear. Sometimes the medications work for a while and then they stop. Sometimes they only help enough to take "the edge off." Other times, there are too many side effects and the person has to stop the medication all together. Unfortunately, doctors do not have it all figured out, either. Therefore, we cannot assume the person is still sick because they have not been doing everything they can do to get better.

There is no doubt we really do want to help, because we really do care. All the same, try to imagine if every person you met assumed you were sick or in pain, because you were sitting around doing nothing about it or you did not *want* to improve. If a condition is chronic, this means it is ongoing, and we need to avoid getting frustrated with the sick person when they are not well.

They Need A Better Attitude

Oh, cheer up! Look the bright side!
Hey, try to keep your mind off of it.
Be Positive! Mind over matter!

First of all, we need to realize that our loved one is dealing with more than a personality flaw and an inability to create *mind over matter.* "One of the greatest human challenges is found in the demands of an illness that becomes ruthlessly ongoing and chronic. A chronic illness accompanies every move the individual makes. It casts a constant pall over thoughts and actions."[2]

Second, our loved one is dealing with losses, changes, new limitations and inability to participate in their favorite activities. This can cause an enormous amount of discouragement and despair. "Chronic medical illness demands continuous coping and a flexible range of responses, from minimal life change to severe disruption of daily activities."[3]

Third, unlike illnesses that come and go, "Chronic illnesses are different. They do not follow the predictable path from warning signs to recovery"[4] When the body is dealing with constant symptoms, it can actually change the entire chemistry of the system. Overcoming moodiness or depression takes more than the person's desire to be happy. For example, my pain management specialist explained to me how there are actual physiological responses to my condition that I cannot simply "will" away. Therefore, telling our friend or family member to merely, "think healthy thoughts" or use "mind over matter" is not only an uninformed response, but also devastating to our loved ones!

When we tell our loved ones they need a positive attitude, we are actually implying they do not have a good attitude or that it is not *good* enough. As we have seen, it takes an enormous amount of fortitude to live with an ongoing illness. In actuality, our loved ones are displaying immeasurable perseverance and positive attitude, considering the psychological and physical obstacles they are up against. Let us try acknowledging how incredible they are for their perseverance and efforts to enjoy life. After all, we know that when most people are sick for more than a week, they certainly do not have the best attitude. What's more, they even have the luxury of knowing it is going to come to an end!

They Must Not Understand God's Healing Power

Why are you still suffering?
Don't you know that God can heal you?
If He can heal my friend, He can heal you!

God *can* heal and God *does* heal! What good news! Praise the Lord! However, "Many Christians misinterpret Jesus' promise of the 'abundant life' (John 10:10) to mean perfect health, a comfortable lifestyle, constant happiness, full realization of your dreams, and instant relief from problems through faith and prayer. In a word, they expect the Christian life to be easy. They expect heaven on earth."[5]

Because of this, it is easy to believe our loved ones must not understand who God is since they have not been healed. Essentially, we are thinking the chronically ill must not know God like we do, since they are still sick. Besides, to claim they should have been healed, tells them we think they are sick because they lack hope and belief in God's power. Regrettably, this degrades a person's relationship with God when we pronounce that they are ill because they do not grasp who He is.

Imagine being constantly bombarded by well-meaning brothers and sisters, insisting you have to listen to a tape or read a book by someone who proclaims God can heal you! Unless our loved ones are not believers or we know for a fact that they do not have any faith at all, we should not jump to the conclusion that they need to read a book to know this. Our loved ones do not need to be inspired or coached into believing they can be healed. They should already know this, because they have the best book of all and that is the Bible, which is by the only true Healer, who is Jesus.

It can be encouraging; in fact, to hear how others were healed and relieved of their pain and many times it gives hope! What a time to rejoice and celebrate! On the other hand, it can be aggravating for a person when every believer they meet feels compelled to inform them of how someone else was healed, as if they must not realize that God is capable. That may make them feel as if others are questioning their faith by asking, "Why are you still suffering? Don't you understand that God can heal you, too?"

Finally, we cannot assume that because someone is still suffering, they must not have prayed for healing. Nor can we deduce that they misunderstand or under appreciate God's healing power. Moreover, we cannot assume our loved ones failed to fully expect, with great faith, to receive God's healing when they prayed.

They Must Be Hiding A Sin

Since you have not been healed, you must be in sin.
What sin are you hiding?

It is so tempting to jump to the conclusion that people who contend with a lingering illness must be to blame. When we can find a reason why their pain continues, then we can simply point it out so they can change what they are doing and get better. It seems like the best solution for everyone, because now they can stop suffering. Even more, since we have the answers, we can be confident it will not ever happen to us. Despite what we may think, this is not only harmful, but it can also be utterly devastating when our answer is that our loved one must be in sin or being punished for a sin.

Should sin be considered as a source? Of course! We all need to look into our own hearts and lives and ask for God's discernment. Everyone has sinned and we all "fall short of the glory of God" (Romans 3: 23). In addition, continuing in sin (1 John 3:6) harboring un-confessed sin or un-forgiveness (Matt 9:6), can greatly affect our bodies, minds and souls. Our guilt, uneasiness and shame can cause us both physical and emotional "dis-ease." Most of all, it separates us from intimacy with God and His will.

The sad part is that often people living with illness are not *approached* about sin; they are *accused*. First, we must keep in mind that those with disabilities have probably been approached many, many times. If they have been ill for several years, think of how often they may have been spoken to in regards to this issue. This can be a very touchy and hurtful subject. Second, we should probably only address this issue if we have an established relationship with the person and feel so led while in prayer with them. This must only be done in private, with love and without accusation. It is also in agreement with Romans 8:1 which says, "Therefore there is no condemnation for those who are in Christ Jesus." Third, we must understand that whether or not there is sin in the person's life, God is not required to heal us because we asked. Even if we confess our sin, that does not guarantee God will remove the illness. Fourth, let us dismiss the possibility when they have expressed they are not in sin.

In all, we need to realize that sin is not the only reason for the existence of illness, pain and difficulties in this life. This earth was not meant to be home for us and it is not trouble-free! Sometimes we suffer due to the simple result of this fallen world and our mortal bodies. Sometimes it is a consequence of our actions or the actions of others. Other times, God allows us to go through a trial for our own growth and even for His glory.

They Must Not Have Enough Faith

God can heal you, ya know?
If you had enough faith, you would be healed.
God would heal you if you really wanted Him to.

As stated in the previous chapter, it is so easy to assign blame to those who are suffering. If we do not think that a hidden sin is involved, we often conclude a chronically ill person must lack the faith required for God to heal them.

First of all, God *gives* us all a measure of faith; we do not get it from ourselves. "For by the grace given me I say to every one of you: Do not think of yourself more highly than you ought, but rather think of yourself with sober judgment, in accordance with the measure of faith God has given you" (Rom 12:3). Furthermore, He does not require us to have "enough" faith, because He said it only takes the "…faith as small as a mustard seed" (Matt 17:20) to move a mountain. It does not say the faith of a giant, but the faith of a tiny mustard seed. This seed is smaller than other seeds, but grows into a tree (Matt 13:32). Even so, He does not wait until we have the faith of the tree, but of the little mustard seed.

Second, Jesus taught that it was not the blind man's lack of faith that hindered his being healed. Rather, he was born blind "…so that the work of God might be displayed in his life" (John 9:3). What's more, it clearly was not unbelief that brought Job's sickness on him (Job 1:1). No! Job showed he had a profound faith, in that he continued to serve God even though he had yet to be healed. Living out faith means praising and worshipping God despite adversity; it means asking for God's healing and grace, but knowing that His will is what is best, even when we do not understand. "Trust in the LORD with all of your heart and lean not on your own understanding; in all your ways acknowledge Him, and He will make your paths straight" (Prov 3:5 & 6).

Third, we often think when someone is suffering, that it is a sign they *lack* faith. Quite the opposite it is when our lives are *unchallenged* that we lack faith. Renowned preacher and author, Charles Spurgeon elaborated, "Faith untried may be true faith, but it is sure to be little faith. It is likely to remain stunted as long as it is without trials. Faith never prospers as well as when all things are against her."[6] Therefore, when a person's life is without great suffering, what faith is required of them to trust the Lord?

Oh, what faith is required of us to trust the Lord in the midst of adversity! "Problems force us to look to God and depend on him instead of ourselves. You'll never know that God is all you need until God is all you've got."[2] Those with disabilities, illnesses and injuries must fully rely on God, rather than in themselves. They do not always understand why they have to live with these limitations, but many still give God the glory and praise despite their circumstances. They know the Bible tells us that God is in control, so many continue to live not always knowing *why*, but hopeful in His purpose. This is *untold* faith many will never comprehend unless they suffer greatly and for an extended period of time.

Part Two Summary

Overall, these reactions are quite natural. We are not conditioned to understand how someone who looks perfectly able might not be. The enormity of accepting that our loved one has a serious condition is terrifying, so we protect ourselves by remaining in denial. We may even refuse to acknowledge the illness, thinking that if we pretend it is not there that somehow it will go away.

In all honesty, we really do believe what our loved one is going through is very real, difficult and devastating. Dealing with the actual magnitude of what has happened; the losses and the unknown future can seem consuming. Accordingly, we often use our defense mechanisms to remain in denial and try to down play the circumstances, while we wait for something to fix it. "Coping is blocked; behavioral adaptations become non-existent or dysfunctional as the family waits and wishes for a miracle to put things right again."[8]

We want so much for our loved ones to be okay, so we try desperately to believe that it is really *not that bad*. Unfortunately, we often end up trivializing what they are going through and trying to force them to say their life has been unaffected. As a result, when we really want to show our deepest compassion, we think we have to prove somehow that we can empathize. Still, we cannot act as if our struggle with a common cold compares to an ongoing, debilitating condition. As writer Paul Borthwick put it, "Acute pain is a night in jail. Chronic pain is a long-term prison sentence without parole."[9]

The hardest part about trying to console a loved one, is trying to do so without feeling pressured to come up with an instant solution. We hate to see our loved one suffer, so we stumble to find the words to make all of the hurt go away. This usually leads to coming up with pat answers that really will not work and do not make sense. Furthermore, it could make her feel like we think she has not even made any effort to improve her condition.

So, what does this all mean? Does it mean that we need to keep a list with us of what not to say, so we can tiptoe around our loved one? No! The purpose of Part Two was to help us understand why someone who is ill may get frustrated with us. If we can grasp an understanding of how our words can impact those we love, hopefully we will have the desire to be mindful of our words and actions! We must learn to be considerate of their situation and resist flippant blame for their condition.

"The trick, I guess, is to learn how to think before you speak. Most adults have to learn to do this at work and with their families. If you think it might hurt someone - don't say it. It's hard to do - but like everything else in life, practice makes perfect" Sue Klaus, an audiologist living with Chronic Fatigue Syndrome said. "Would you feel less pressure if you didn't have to say anything at all? Then relax, because sometimes the less you say the better...the action of listening instead of persisting in idle chatter can mean so much more to someone..."[10]

If you have said any of these things listed previously to your loved one, do not become immobilized by guilt! It is not too late! Read on to find out how you can truly be a source of support and fortification! Get together with your friend or family member and tell them you want to work harder at listening and encouraging them. Admit that you responded in a way that you now realize may have been hurtful - *and ask for forgiveness.*

Part Three

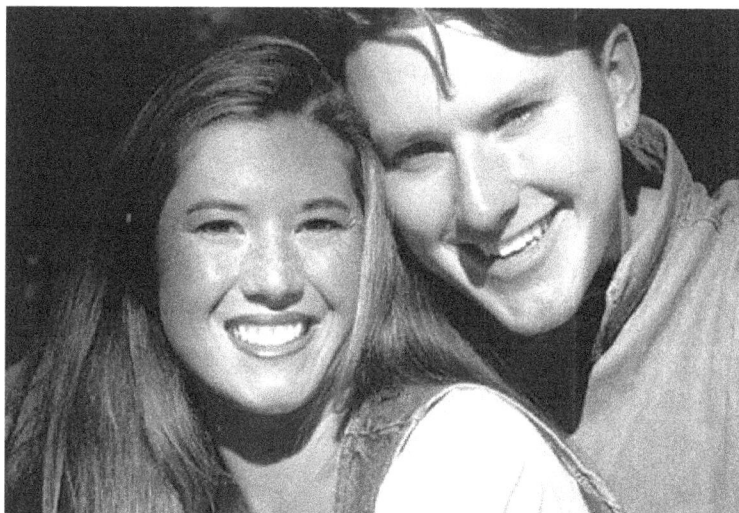

Discovering Some
Encouraging Steps

Rejoice with those who rejoice, and weep with those who weep. Be of the same mind toward one another; do not be haughty in mind, but associate with the lowly.
Do not be wise in your own estimation.

Romans 12: 15 & 16 NASB

Chapter Seven
Knowing the Individual Situation

People with chronic illness and pain are not all the same. In order to be a true sense of support, it is important to remember there are different stages and levels of limitations for each person. It is vital to know how the illness has affected our loved ones, in order to know how to best to encourage them. Some are still able to work, with few restrictions; some work, but it is all they can do to get through the day; some struggle to work part-time; some cannot work at all; some "work" at trying to make meals, go to the doctor or take a shower.

"Become somewhat educated on his illness. Ask him if he'd mind answering some of your questions. Remember, because you've read a book doesn't mean that you know how he is feeling physically or emotionally"[1] Copen recommended. Those with chronic conditions will welcome your questions, as long as you are *asking questions about their illness"* and you are not *"questioning their illness."* Here are some basic levels of severity in illness and pain and how they might manifest:

Level 1: Many people have mild symptoms and are still able to function throughout the day with maybe a few limitations; they will have mostly good days and a few bad days when they overdo, do not watch their diet or do not take their medications.

Level 2: Most have mild-moderate symptoms and with some limitations are still able to function for the most part. Their symptoms may come and go or they may be manageable most of the time, but they still face not being able to "do everything" they want to do. They will have mostly good days and some bad days.

Level 3: Others have moderate-severe symptoms and have to make big adjustments in their lives; it takes all they have to keep a part-time job and/or raise their children. They push themselves all day at work or at home and rarely find energy to have fun. Many have to give up their careers, because the stress and physical demands were unobtainable or they made the person worse. They will have many bad days and fewer good days.

Level4: Some have severe-unbearable symptoms and struggle to keep some sense of their lives; they spend all day trying to perform daily tasks like laundry, cooking a meal or grocery shopping. Others in this category are so ill that their daily goals of showering, going to the doctor or answering some phone calls are an overwhelming battle to obtain. They will have mostly horrible-horrific days and some do not have any good days at all.

Therefore, it is very important to know what level of symptoms and frequency your loved one is experiencing, in order to truly know how to be an encouragement. Even people with the same diagnosis do not have an equal level of symptoms. Because your cousin Jeff is doing great and still able to work with his Multiple Sclerosis, does not mean your friend Sarah, with the same illness, is able to do the same.

In Part Two, we discovered that we cannot make a visual diagnosis of how someone "feels" by how they "look." We also addressed our natural responses to continuing health conditions, taking a look at comments made when we are reacting to these difficult situations and found out why they can be hurtful. We have been able to see how remaining in denial, trivializing their circumstances and refusing to acknowledge the truth can cause them to feel like we do not believe them.

Moreover, we have learned how claiming or even insinuating that our loved one does not have enough faith, is in sin or does not understand God's healing power, can crush the very person we should be admiring for their display of true faith and dependence on God!

In the following four chapters, we will provide steps to encouraging someone living with an illness, injury or disability. In doing this, we will give some examples of what to say and explain why these points are so important.

Chapter Eight
Validate and Grieve

The first step in ministering to someone with a chronic condition is for us to validate their situation and allow them to grieve their losses.

Allow Them to LOOK Good

You sure look nice today! Wow! Don't you look handsome?
That outfit looks really good on you!

It says in the book of John, "Stop judging by mere appearances, and make a right judgment" (John 7:24). Instead, value each person individually, because they are made in God's own image (Gen 1:27).

Because a person who is sick with a disease or disorder does not always look ill or in pain to others, we often conclude it either must not be true or it cannot be that bad. Lisa, a lady with MS wrote, "People always say, 'you don't look like you're sick!' I get so tired of hearing that."[1] This makes our loved one feel as if we seem to be calling them a liar.

It is devastating when we refuse to believe what we cannot see with our own eyes. We question their character and integrity when we tell them what they are saying cannot be true, because we cannot see it. Now, they not only have their disorder to contend with, but also our disbelief of them. This has the appearance that we have no idea what they are going through.

On the other hand, we should not expect to *see* a dysfunction that lives in the organs, blood, bones and nervous system. Therefore, we do not have to "see it" to "believe it!" If we want to know how someone is doing or feeling, we can simply ask. When they give us the answer, we must believe. If we want to remark on how great they look, without presuming it must mean they are feeling good - go ahead! "It's okay to say it, but understand that looking good doesn't necessarily mean your loved one feels good."[2] Everyone wants to look his or her best and everyone enjoys a compliment!

If we refuse to believe there is a race being run, how can we commend them for the perseverance to keep running? If we refuse to acknowledge the hurdles even exist, how can we see their strength and determination to battle obstacles? Let us take a moment to see the marathon at hand, so we can be the ones handing them water and cheering them on!

Acknowledge the Illness or Injury

Wow! I had no idea you were in such pain.
I may not fully understand, but I believe you and I believe in you.
It must be so hard to be sick so much.

It is plain dreadful to see another person hurting! Our natural instinct is to protect the ones we love and ourselves. Nevertheless, we have seen how that can flounder into painful inferences. "It is often not only the disease itself that is painful, but also the emotional effects of having the illness discounted, having one's respectability and judgment questioned, and dealing with the criticisms of others. It is extremely necessary for the person with chronic illness to feel that his disease is validated, even by people that he doesn't know."[3]

I know it is so hard to do, but we must acknowledge the illness exists and is real. We must stop questioning our loved ones' integrity and start showing them that we not only *believe* them, but we also believe *in* them. We should become educated on their condition by asking them where we can get some information and most of all by discussing their personal experiences with them.

Acknowledging their illness and its impact on their lives will help to free them from the burden of having to convince us of what they are going through! Additionally, "with this cognitive awareness, [we] can more easily begin the coping and grieving processes, and ultimately come to some level of understanding about their situation."[4]

This can actually bring everyone together to form a troop to battle the war at hand. "Like an intruder, chronic illness sneaks into your house unexpectedly and robs valuable items from everyone who lives there," described Gregg Piburn, author and husband of a woman who lives with chronic illness. "I find value in personifying the illness because it creates an impetus to fight back. We go to war against the intruder."[5]

Acknowledge Their Losses

I am so sorry you can't work anymore.
I can't imagine what you have been through.
It must be so hard not to be able to that.

Many caregivers, family members and friends think if they minimize the situation or tell their friend "it is not that bad," the illness or pain will be easier to deal with. On the contrary, that will only lead to hurt and resentment. Alternatively, when we acknowledge what they have been through, lost and are still facing, they will gain a new strength, knowing we are there to fight the battle with them!

It is imperative that we confirm their loss as real, before we can proceed to the next steps to grief, then coping and adapting. When we address the situation, we also recognize it as a validated loss, so that "…families will be better able to construct a new meaning of their situation and move on with their lives…"[6]

The losses surrounding a limiting condition have a great impact on everyone involved. "The losses go far beyond the former healthy body; they often include loss of employment, loss of income, loss of intellectual acuity, loss of former expectations, loss of social life, and so on" writer Susan Dion declared. "Indeed, the illness results in the loss of varied parts of the self."[7] Therefore, we must allow them to grieve what they can no longer do, by sitting, listening and being there for them.

The Bible commands us to "Carry each other's burdens, and in this way you will fulfill the law of Christ" (Gal 6:2). We must remember your brother in bondage as if you are bound with them (Heb 13:3). Without completing this step we can, "[predict] symptoms such as depression, anxiety, loss of mastery, hopelessness, and conflict, all of which erode couple and family relationships."[8]

Acknowledge Their Desire to Do More

Please don't feel pressured to help; I know that being here is difficult enough.
I know you would love to do so much more,
I am so sorry you can't!

It is SO frustrating and heartbreaking for them to not be able to participate in ministry, functions, groups, studies and activities, as they would like to! Many times, before their illness, they were very involved with committees, the choir and the youth. Now it may be all they can do to make it to church or a Bible study. They get aggravated with both themselves and their inability to do what they want to do and feel guilty for not being able to help. It is reassuring when we let our loved ones know we acknowledge their dilemma and relieve them of the pressure put upon them not only by others, but by themselves.

Chapter Nine
Show Admiration

The second step to ministering to someone with a chronic condition is for us to show admiration for him or her.

Admire Their Faith

I admire your love for God, in the midst of your circumstances!
It's amazing how you continue to praise God, despite your pain.
Your life is a real testimony of faith!

Although people who have chronic conditions are often looked upon as *lacking* faith, the opposite is often true. Try to imagine losing your career, ability to take your children places, care for your garden, participate in your beloved hobbies, cook, clean or enjoy activities you have always loved. What would you do?

"...it is one thing to love the ways of the Lord when all is fair and quite another to cleave to them under all discouragements and difficulties. Where do you stand? Is your heart fixed on Jesus?" Spurgeon challenged. "Have you counted the cost, and are you solemnly ready to suffer all worldly loss for the Master's sake? Worldly treasures are not to be compared with the glory to be revealed."[1]

As noted before, many who suffer from chronic illness and pain are told that their conditions are a sign that they are lacking faith. They are often viewed as being uncertain of God's power, since they are still sick. But the Lord knows it takes true faith to continue through the storms! "No faith is so precious as that which lives and triumphs in adversity."[2]

It takes untiring faith to live with physical obstacles and losses! Believers with chronic conditions have chosen to praise the Lord despite their constant battles with pain, loss and an uncertain future. They have chosen to look to God for their every strength and He gives them the grace and power to do so. God wants all of His children to be fully reliant upon Him. "Your most profound and intimate experiences of worship will likely be in your darkest days – when your heart is broken, when you feel abandoned, when you're out of options, when the pain is great..."[3] With their wounded bodies and minds, those who are suffering are right where God wants us all: depending on Him for our every need - and that is living a life of true faith!

Job continued to have faith in God, even though his wife told him to turn from this God who would not heal him. He knew the Lord had the power to heal him and he continued to worship God even though he was still afflicted. Job said, "Though he slay me, yet will I hope in him" (Job 13:15a). Job fully trusted in God, His will and His power to heal him, even though he was still suffering. He had unfathomable faith in God, despite his circumstances; he knew God was hearing his case and that God was in control. And, that is *true faith!*

Let us lift our loved ones up, by recognizing what trust in God's plan it takes to live in their situation! We can do this by showing our admiration for them and our awe for God's grace to provide their sustenance. We can assure our loved ones that the Lord's strength is evident in him or her and that their life is a living example of *true faith*.

Acknowledge Their Perseverance

It amazes me how you keep fighting!
I don't know if I would be as strong if I were in your position.
I can't believe how much you have done to get your health back!

We often question our loved ones' desire to recuperate when the illness continues for a long period of time. What we fail to realize is that they have probably not only researched their options again and again, but they have gone from doctor to doctor, taken dozens of medications, had several procedures and have even sought alternative help.

The truth is if our friends or family members are crying and telling us that they cannot stand being sick, it should be obvious they are not being lazy. People who are slacking do not usually protest their situations, express grief over their losses and plead to get their lives back. If they are showing frustration for their situation, we can bet they are doing everything they can to get better.

Let us take a closer look to see the incredible fortitude someone with a chronic illness or injury actually does possess! God uses our difficulties to show that He is much bigger than our problems, by giving us purpose and strength to go on. As pastor, Bob Buchanan announced, "Through weakness and suffering and pain and loss and tragedy the grace of God causes us to persevere through afflictions and shows that God is compellingly greater than the affliction."[4]

What a witness we are of God working through our weaknesses and troubles during difficult times! For "Blessed is the man who perseveres under trial, because when he has stood the test, he will receive the crown of life that God has promised to those who love him" (James 1:12).

Acknowledge Their Courage and Attitude

I can't imagine being sick all of the time.
I don't know how you do it. You amaze me.
I can't believe how you keep fighting.

It can be a constant battle to live with an illness. Many with chronic conditions are struggling to get through a day at work or at home with the kids. They do not have energy beyond that to enjoy their hobbies, be involved in the church like they want to be or do their chores. Others push and push themselves all day to make it into the shower, feed the pets or make a meal. Some even feel like their lives are being wasted away spending all of their time going to doctor appointments, straightening out insurance issues, filling out paperwork, trying new medications, doing their therapies and paying medical bills.

No matter how serious or how minor it is, there are limitations and giving up of enjoyable activities. Do not be afraid to praise them for their courage and determination! Commend them for their overall attitude; consider their losses, frustrations and inner physiological rivalry. We can give them such incentive to keep going by doing these things. Then, we will begin to see a huge change in their outlook!

Appreciate Their Efforts to Make it Out of the house

I am so glad you were able to make it! Wow! You made it!
It is so great to see you; I know it is quite a sacrifice for you!

We often think when we see someone who lives with a chronic

condition that it must mean they are feeling *well* since they are out and about. We do not realize that many who are debilitated by illness cannot wait for a good day to get to the grocery store or go to church. Therefore, they must push themselves to get a few things done or to enjoy life, despite their pain. What is more, they will probably pay a high price for that outing for many days to come.

When we assume they are out and about because they are feeling well, we fail to recognize what great determination they have. We prove to them that we probably do not have any idea what mountain they have climbed to get there and how much their symptoms will inflame afterwards. The worst part for them is in knowing that because we assumed they were doing great, we possibly will not be keeping them in prayer. This makes them feel alone in their battle, because we obviously have no idea what they are going through.

Instead, we must show our admiration for their strength and perseverance. After all, we know that if we felt that bad, we would certainly not be out. We should tell them we appreciate their company and acknowledge what it must have taken to get there and the cost it will pose later. Mostly, we need to assure them that we will be in prayer in the coming days as they pay that price.

Not By Sight...82

Chapter Ten
Adjust and Adapt

The third step to ministering to someone with a chronic condition is for us to learn how to adjust and adapt to the new changes.

Do Not Try to Fix Everything

Although I will keep praying for a miracle, I love you the way you are. Even though you cannot do all of the things you used to do, you are still very valuable to those who know you.

Often, we bombard our loved ones with information about medications, vitamins and articles, etc. We must keep in mind that everyone else is giving them advice as well and that can be overwhelming! "If you want to suggest a cure to me, please don't. It's not because I don't appreciate the thought, and it's not because I don't want to get well" Oberin appealed. "It's because I have had almost every single one of my friends suggest one at one point or another."[1]

It is tough to see a person in distress, so we feel like we have to say the right things to make it all go away. In any case, when we pressure ourselves to come up with a quick fix answer, it usually ends up being something trite or unfounded. After all, if the person has had the illness for 5 years, the answer must not be as simple as we would like to think it is. Let's face it! We are probably not going to think of a solution in 5 minutes that they have not thought of in 5 years!

In addition, when we are always jumping to a quick fix solution, we attempt to avoid all conversation regarding the situation. By doing this, we hope that the answer will provide a means to make the issue go away. "The problem is that we are often in so much of a hurry to fix things that we don't have time to sympathize with people."[2]

Unfortunately, we then fail to work through the proper steps of grieving and coping, which can lead to depression, frustration, isolation and resentment for everyone involved. Conversely, "Those not insistent on…finding perfect solutions to every problem can live with ambiguous losses without negative effects to themselves or the patient."[3]

To be supportive, we must meet the person *right where they are* and minister to their needs. The Bible says we should come along side those who are hurting and cry *with* them. It does not say that we need to make them *stop* crying; it tells us to hold their hand and *mourn with* them. "Rejoice with those who rejoice; mourn with those who mourn. Live in harmony with one another. Do not be proud, but be willing to associate with people of low position. Do not be conceited" (Rom 12: 15 & 16).

For that reason, the best thing to do is to listen, learn and discuss the situation, rather than feeling as if we have to say something that will make it suddenly disappear. It brings great joy to our loved one, when a fellow believer hears with compassion, allows expression of their thoughts and comes along side of them to offer a shoulder, without a word of blame, accusation or need to fix it. "Blessed are the merciful, for they will be shown mercy" (Matt 5:7). A kind, loving ear can do wonders for the heart.

Our friends or family members simply want to know they are

valuable to us, just as they are, even when they are broken and not at their full potential. They want to know we are willing to weep with them over their losses. Moreover, they do not want to feel like we will only accept them if they are repaired and whole again. This will not cause them to stop fighting, because they want their health back as much or more than we do and they are doing everything they can to get it! They do not want to give up on hope, an answer or a miracle either. In the meantime, we must be careful not to ignore what they are going through right now.

Respect Their Limitations

If this is too much for you, let me know.
Hey, I would love for you to come over Friday night;
but if you can't, I'll understand.

Having unwanted limitations is discouraging to say the least. The last thing anyone wants is to lose parts of their lives that make them happy and bring them joy. Even so, when a person experiences recurrent limitations, they must learn to set boundaries. With time, they will discover that the price of failing to stay within those boundaries will most likely cause them to worsen and have to give up even more afterwards.

Most people know what it is like to become tired after helping at church or with a family get together. For our brother or sister, this can cause them to be much more than simply tired. Their condition could flare up and exacerbate into severe pain, physiological imbalance, unbearable fatigue or even depression for several days or even weeks from the seemingly simple activity. "Respect her limitations and be sensitive to them. Don't say, 'A little walk might do you some good' or 'No pain, no gain!'"[4]

We must also remember that if a person has to say "no" to an activity that it does not mean they do not *want* to go! If they say they *can't*, they mean they *can't*. It does not mean they don't *want* to. In fact, they *despise* having to say "no" and being forced to give up another part of their lives! It tears them up inside when they have to miss out on another activity. If we argue with them when they are physically unable to participate, they will not only have to contend with being discouraged about missing the event, but also realizing we think they are choosing not to go and using the illness as an excuse.

Do not question how they how they can do something one day, but not on another. Often "…the patient's condition ebbs and flows, some days able to be as they always were before the illness, other times, preoccupied with pain and exhaustion."[5] They may even step out of what they should be doing once in a while, but that does not mean they can do that all of the time. "Only she knows her limits and they will likely change from day to day depending on many factors. What she could do yesterday may not be possible today. Don't question that."[6]

Does this mean we should not ask them to go places with us, since they usually say, "no?" We sure hope not! When people stop asking, they think we have given up on them and that makes them feel even more left out and isolated! Of course, if they tell us they are no longer able to do a certain thing, let us not keep asking them to do it! Otherwise, as long as we are willing to accept hearing "no" once in a while or even most of the time, we need to keep asking!

Not By Sight…86

Make Modifications

I would love to pick up groceries for you on my way home.
Let's sit down and make a list of the family chores.
Each of us is going to pitch in more from now on.

Once we acknowledge limitations, we can learn to make the proper adaptations. Boss suggested for therapists to "…set the stage for conversations among family member of several generations until the group reaches some measure of consensus about what has been irretrievably lost, as well as how to enjoy the capabilities the ill person still has."[7]

In order to make necessary adjustments, we need to reorganize the family responsibilities and clarify our expectations. First, we must make a list of what our loved one can no longer do or should no longer be doing, for the best interest of their well-being. Second, we need to figure out a way to get these things done, by letting family and friends sign up for a chore or hiring someone. Third, we need to make a list of those things they would like to try to do, but may or may not be able to complete them regularly. Forth, we need to make a back-up plan or assign an "understudy" for the duties they may be unable to do all of the time. "As they begin seeing the ill person as still in the family, but in a new way, the family boundaries and roles become clearer. As perceptions are shared, the immobilized system begins to shift and adapt."[8]

Therefore, as we make clear our expectations of our loved one and everyone else in the support system, we can go from resentment of the person, to understanding, to adjusting and coping. We can stop being frustrated with what the person can no longer do, when we finally accept it as plain reality. We can still pray for a miracle or a cure, but in the meantime it is imperative that we adapt to what we are dealing with right now!

Find Joy

Let's make a list of fun things the family can still do.
I know you can't go skiing anymore,
but maybe we can still spend time doing something else.

So much of the focus with chronic conditions is on the things they can no longer do. While we are making lists of things our loved one cannot manage, let's also make a list of the things they think they *can* do with family and friends that is fun and enjoyable! There are still ways to spend time together, if everyone chips in to make them happen. It could be anything from camping to watching a video or from taking a drive to listening to music.

First, make a list of the big impact things that our loved one would like to try, like a vacation or boat ride. Second, we can make a list of medium impact activities like playing a game or going out to a movie that we know could be difficult, but possible. Third, we should make a list of low impact enjoyments, such as having someone in the family read from a book or sitting outside on a nice evening.

Now, we have to remember that how often they will be able to do these and even if they will be able to do them at all needs to be left open! As a result, "...the healthy family member with more resilience and leeway must take the lead in adapting to fluctuating absence and presence, a situation that may not go away."[9] What's more, often our loved one forgoes enjoyable activities, because it is all they can do to get their daily tasks accomplished. Thus, we need to agree that our loved one's usual responsibilities and chores will have to be claimed by family, friends or by other means so that they can trade the tasks for the activity.

Chapter Eleven
Cope and Support

The fourth step to ministering to someone with a chronic condition is for us to learn how to cope with it and be supportive.

Know What to Ask

How are you doing? So, what is really going on?
Honestly, how are you?

We might not realize that people living with chronic illness do not expect us to always stop to hear all of their problems. There are many times when asking, "How are you doing?" is used as a greeting in passing and many answer with a quick, "Fine!" When someone really wants to know how I am, I do prefer to be asked, "How are you doing?" versus being asked, "How are you feeling?" The former question allows me to answer according to my *spiritual* and *emotional* well-being, not my physical state. Usually I can answer with a positive response, as it relates to how I am dealing with life, being sick and the obstacles I face.

On the other hand being asked, "How are you feeling?" deals directly with the physical circumstances. For those who have many good days, it is nice when they can respond with, "I'm feeling well today!" However, for those whose symptoms rarely or never remit, it can be exasperating to always have to answer, "Not good." There is no point in asking someone who is sick or in terrible pain most or all of the time, how he or she is feeling! Personally, when the same people keep asking me this, I feel like pleading, "I don't feel good! I haven't felt good for over 15 years! So, please stop asking." We think it is rude not to ask, but always asking will only make them realize that we do not understand their situation.

When we are truly interested in knowing how they are doing and feeling, we should simply sit down with them to ask. Lorden examined, "I have a couple of wonderful friends who ask me 'how are you?' twice. The first time I respond like everyone else. Then they say, 'okay, now how are you *really*?' Then I feel comforted, knowing they are truly interested and prepared to listen."[1]

Allow Them to Be Honest

It is okay to be honest with me.
I really wish I knew how to help.
Gosh, I don't know how to respond.

First, we must make sure that when we do ask someone how they are feeling or how they are doing, that we are willing to hear the truth. It is imperative that we allow them to be honest with us. "Chronic illness presents a variety of challenges to relationships at a time when they are needed the most."[2] Thus, we need to allow them to vent their concerns, fears and even anger.

We cannot urge them to bottle it up, by expecting them to always be okay with what they are going through. When they need a shoulder, we must be there for them and willing to cry with them. "Once strong and self-confident people may feel inadequate and unlovable due to lack of productivity, inability to work or engage in other activities, discouragement about recovery, coping with debilitating pain and fatigue on a long-term basis, and so much more."[3]

Second, have you ever sat there with your mind scrambling for the right words to make everything better? It is okay to admit that we do not know what to say or how to react. We do not have to feel pressured to come up with a quick answer; instead we need to resist the urge to even try. Unless you are a doctor, pastor, lawyer or counselor, they are probably not looking for answers from you anyway.

So many people think they have to produce an instant solution, but that leads to pat, careless, inappropriate suggestions that are hurtful. "In real fellowship people experience sympathy. Sympathy is not giving advice or offering quick, cosmetic help; sympathy is entering in and sharing the pain of others."[4] We should try listening, acknowledging what they are telling us and commending them for their perseverance. We will be amazed at the positive response!

Third, we know it is difficult for our loved one to live with this, but it is difficult for those around them as well! "Understand that chronic illness impacts the person's 'healthy' loved ones as well" Piburn commented about his struggle with his wife's condition. "I know Sherrie's experience with The Intruder has been much tougher than mine. But having Sherrie realize it was tough on the rest of us, too, helped us band together against a common enemy, The Intruder. We became allies rather than competitors."[5]

Appreciate Our Own Health

I really take my health for granted. You make me appreciate being able to do things I usually think of as chores.

We have all heard the saying, "You don't know what you've got until it's gone!" Once a person living with an illness has lost some or many of the activities they used to enjoy, they realize that if they could have their lives back the way they were, they would be SO much more appreciative of what they had! Thus, it is rewarding for them to see others realize this, while still able to accomplish so much and live a full, active life. "It is wise to learn from experience, it is wiser to learn from the experiences of others."[6] If they can be one thing, let them be a reminder to appreciate your health and be thankful for being able to do those things taken for granted every day.

Pray for Them

When you feel all alone, remember I am praying for you. I will pray for God's strength to sustain you.

It is consoling to know others are praying on our behalf, because it is God alone who sustains us. To know our friends and family are keeping us lifted up to our Lord is such a comfort. When we offer prayer, it is good to ask *how* we can pray, instead of *if* we can pray. This lets others know we are interested in the details of their needs and that we are willing to hear about them.

When praying for someone with a chronic condition, we need to be mindful not to be fixated on healing. I am not saying we should not pray for healing, a cure or a miracle! We can petition the Lord for healing daily if we want to! Yet, our focus must be for God's will because, "This is the confidence we have in approaching God: that if we ask anything according to his will, he hears us" (1 John 5:14). We also must be patient and full of thanks for what He has already done, as we give our request, "Do not be anxious about anything, but in everything, by prayer and petition, with thanksgiving, present your requests to God" (Phil 4:6).

Our loved one mourns the loss of parts of their life and freedom; he or she wants to be healed more than we can begin to imagine! However, when healing does not occur, they can become very discouraged and depressed. Therefore, when we pray for healing, we must be very   careful not to: 1) Blame them if healing does not occur, 2) Make them feel as if they have to be healed or they must not have a right relationship with God, 3) Make them feel pressured to tell us they are better (if they are not) after we have prayed.

In all, it is very important that we do not strive for healing as the only answer to our requests. It only creates more guilt and frustration when God says, "No." Most of all, we do not want to put up barriers against God's ultimate purpose and block their ability to see how He might be working in them right now as they are!

As we wait on God, we should also pray for strength, peace and joy amidst the suffering. "And the peace of God, which transcends all understanding, will guard your hearts and your minds in Christ Jesus" (Phil 4:7). The bottom line is that God is God and only He knows what is best for us! Trusting God means we are putting our lives in *His* hands. When we pray for His will, we put our confidence in Him to do what *He* thinks is best for our lives. Besides, we must understand that God, "…usually prefers to work through people rather than perform miracles, so that we will depend on each other for fellowship."[7] Maybe we are the answer to our own prayer for them! We should stop insisting God create a miracle and *be one!*

Part Three Summary

As believers, we are accountable to be compassionate and loving! Paul said, "Therefore, as God's chosen people, holy and dearly loved, clothe yourselves with compassion, kindness, humility, gentleness and patience" (Col 3:12).

We do not need to blurt out platitudes because, "He who answers before listening- that is his folly and his shame" (Prov 18:13). Furthermore, we certainly should not put blame upon them and tear down the very thing that keeps them going – their faith and relationship with the Lord.

As an alternative, we should follow the proper steps of loss, so we can *all* adapt and cope in a healthy way. We must acknowledge their situation, make modifications, show them our admiration and be there for support. We also must pray with them for strength and peace that comes solely from our Lord. This is the *only* way that we can address the issue at hand, make adjustments and find joy despite the circumstances!

When we are willing to show our support with compassion, we will find them gaining determination from our belief in them. When we acknowledge the mountain they are climbing and praise them for their courage, we will witness a transformation in their outlook. Let us come along side of them to pray for strength, perseverance and peace as we wait on the Lord in His will.

Part Four

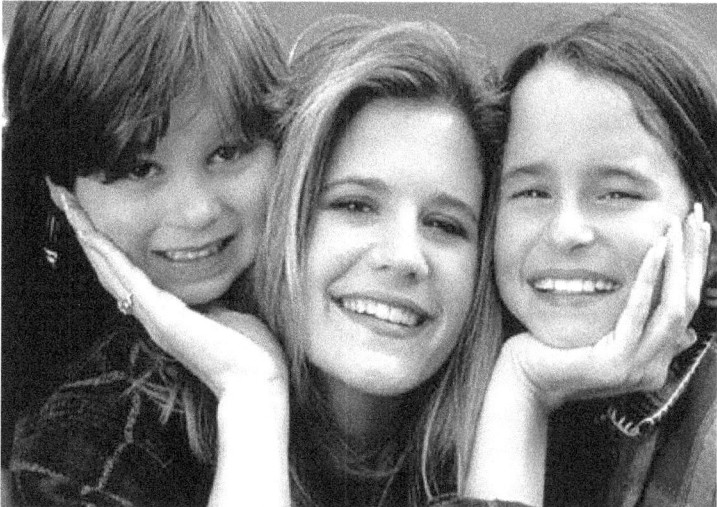

Bringing It All
Together In Love

*So, as those who have been chosen of God,
holy and beloved, put on a heart of
compassion, kindness, humility,
gentleness and patience.*

Colossians 3: 12 NASB

Chapter Twelve
The Problem

We are a world of busy schedules and quick fixes. We fill our day timers up to the brim with so many activities that we do not have a minute to spare. If we find ourselves ill, we postpone going to the doctor because we really do not have the time. If it gets bad enough, we will finally go to plea to them for a quick cure. Most walk out with a prescription and instructions to end the misery within a few days or a couple of weeks.

As a result, how do we respond when we meet someone who has been ill or in pain for several months or even several years? Do we assume they must not be seeking help? After all, we believe that if they would go to the doctor, they would get better too. Thus, when we find out they have already been to the doctor, do we assume they must not have followed the directions, they did not go to the right doctor or they must not want to get better?

What if we are believers? How do we respond? Do we understand that God is in control and stand by this person with love, prayer and compassion? Or do we fault our loved one and blame the illness on sin, lack of faith or failure to say the right words and perform the right rituals?

Dealing with tragedy is tough - none of us wants to face it! We often try to find the words, solutions and Scriptures that will make it "all go away." We cannot imagine going through that ourselves, it is way too much to comprehend. Therefore we often attempt to minimize the situation and pretend that it either does not exist or that "it is not really that bad."

We honestly believe we are doing the right thing, saying the right thing, being positive and supportive! So, we are puzzled when we try to help and are met with frustration or what seems to be resistance to our suggestions. All too often, we find our relationship with our loved one strained and at an impasse. We become unable to communicate on common ground, as each cannot understand the other and become frustrated and confused.

Chapter Thirteen
The Solution

The biggest blockade people have is worrying about what to say. Healthy people living in relationship to someone with chronic illness or disability think they have to talk about the illness or come up with solutions. But, the truth is we do not have to feel pressured to always address the illness, because our friend or family member will not always want to talk about it either. We are not expected to have the answers; in fact, he or she might prefer we not even try.

If we do not know what to talk about to someone struggling with illness, we can talk about marriage, kids or favorite movies, the same topics we would talk about with any of our other friends. Or, we can try asking about what kind of work they did or what they studied in college (if they were able to do this before). No, it is not always good to live our lives in the past, but it can be helpful for us to learn about hobbies, skills, talents, past accomplishments and pleasures enjoyed before the illness. It gives us a better sense of who they are, where they are today and can help us realize the scope of their losses and struggles. "One key to courtesy is to understand where people are coming from. Discover their history. When you know what they've been through, you will be more understanding."[1]

Yes, people with chronic conditions are hoping we will try to understand what they are going through. But, they do not expect us to have a *complete* understanding of the enormity of what they have lost, are feeling and are experiencing. "You can try to explain and explain again, by listing your worst symptoms or the many well-documented body-wide abnormalities, or by trying to use metaphors," Livingston exposed. "…but the plain fact is this: no one who hasn't personally suffered from chronic illness can ever be expected fully to understand it."[2]

If we feel our loved ones are constantly complaining or repeatedly telling us how sick they are, it may be they think we do not believe them or appreciate the seriousness of what they are going through. Once we acknowledge their illness, losses and struggles, their attitudes will change! They will shift from struggling for our validation to fighting the problem at hand.

As healthy friends, family members, care givers and encouragers, we need to discover that when we do not validate what the person is going through, but try to deny or play down the situation, minimizing the illness and consequent losses can make our loved one feel as if we are accusing them of being dishonest about the severity of their condition. When we fail to address their very real and legitimate losses, they will only feel even more isolated and alone in their fight for normalcy and understanding.

Instead of telling others they need "snap out of it" or "buck it up," Paul exhorted fellow brothers and sisters to be strong *for* them: "Now we who are strong ought to bear the weaknesses of those without strength and not *just* please ourselves" (Rom 15:1). Jesus said, "…whatever you did not do for one of the least of these, you did not do for me" (Matt 25: 45).

In heaven, God will "...review how you treated other people, particularly those in need. Jesus said the way to love him is to love his family and care for their practical needs."[3] It can be challenging, but we are even required to come up along side our brothers and sisters and cry with them! "Praise be to the God and Father of our Lord Jesus Christ, the Father of compassion and the God of all comfort, who comforts us in all our troubles, so that we can comfort those in any trouble with comfort we ourselves have received from God" (2 Cor 1: 3 & 4).

It saddens me to think that some people feel it is a burden to be my friend. Some people might fear our relationship will be all one-sided with them always having to lift me up. "Healthy friends don't want to bother us with their troubles or needs;" revealed Copen. "...they feel guilty and even embarrassed that they are stressing out over their daughter's new boyfriend or the layoffs at work, when we are wondering if we'll live to see 60. True friends, however, share both the ups and the downs."[4] What I have found is quite the opposite: a few of my good friends know they can come to me when they are having troubles.

I enjoy being there for them and helping them through the tough times. These are my most beloved friendships, the ones where we can mutually share our lives together! Warren put it beautifully, "The deepest, most intense level [of fellowship] is the fellowship of suffering, where we enter into each other's pain and grief and carry each other's burdens."[5]

Let us be sensitive to those who are living with illnesses, injury and disability, for "Blessed is he who has regard for the weak; the LORD delivers him in times of trouble" (Ps 41:1). If we have not been a source of encouragement in this way, we should not worry. It is not too late to love and support our family member or friend! Once we have shown them that we are ready to *believe them* and *believe in* them, our relationship will blossom beyond what we could ever have imagined.

Once we have made it apparent that we support our loved ones, they will be much less apt to seem like complainers who are constantly trying to convince us of their situation. Often the barrier of communication is relieved and the pressure is released, because they will no longer be trying to pound it into our head.

When we take a moment to see the courage of those in a debilitating situation and admire their strength, they will be renewed by our confidence and feel uniquely valued. Suddenly, we will find ourselves enjoying being around this person again. We will know what to say and we will no longer want to avoid them. Moreover, we will be surprised at how much less taxing the relationship is, because we have simply expressed admiration and our belief in them.

Chapter Fourteen
Not By Sight

Last, but certainly not least, let me share one more word about faith. It seems that when we come across someone who is ill or in pain, we may conclude, "that the person must not have enough faith." On the contrary, "Your most profound and intimate experiences of worship will likely be in your darkest days – when your heart is broken, when you feel abandoned, when you're out of options, when the pain is great…"[1]. Therefore, the faith of someone living with an illness, injury or disability can be God focused and the source of all strength!

Fortunately, for many who are living with illnesses, injury and disability, their limitations can be minor and manageable with continuous care and attention. For others, it is all they can do to get through a day at work. Many struggle with not being able to serve at the church with their God given gifts and talents as they would like. Others strive to get to a doctor's appointment or make their meals. Some even lose their careers, hobbies and ability to have children.

Those who are living with illnesses, injury and disability are often forced to juggle their limited efforts, such as knowing if they make dinner means they will not be able to wash their hair. Or going to a doctor's appointment, means they will not be able to make it to a Bible study. Or for those who are still able to work, they know when they get home they will be too exhausted and in pain to do much of anything else. To our amazement, despite whatever they may have lost and struggle through, those who suffer still praise our Lord.

No, they indeed have faith! They have unyielding faith! In fact, they have a more robust faith in God's plan than some who are standing on the outside of their situation. Scottish theologian James S. Stewart asserted, "It is the spectators, the people who are outside, looking at the tragedy, from whose ranks the skeptics come; it is not those who are actually in the arena and who know suffering from the inside."[2]

It takes resolute faith to know that our Lord, Jesus can and will indeed heal - *but in His own time.* A loved one may hope and pray for healing today, believing with all of his or her heart that they will be delivered from their pain. Still, if the answer is "No, not now," then living with that answer is what takes *faith.* "Whenever God says no to your request for relief, remember, 'God is doing what is best for us, training us to live God's holy best' [Heb 12:10b]."[3]

None of us wants to suffer! When He was in the garden, Jesus himself asked for another way, other than to have to endure suffering. The Bible says, "…he fell with his face to the ground and prayed, 'My Father, if it is possible, may this cup be taken from me." Though He requested this from our Lord, he added, "Yet not as I will, but as you will'" (Matt 26: 39).

Later that evening, "He went away a second time and prayed, 'My Father, if it is not possible for this cup to be taken away unless I drink it, may your will be done'" (Matt 26: 42). He then accepted His Father's will, prepared to suffer and gave His life for us all.

Believers living with a chronic condition often develop an

understanding that none of us is God and an assurance that His plan is sovereign. He or she knows they will ultimately receive healing when they are delivered up to Him. To live with such an uncertainty of today, tomorrow and the mortal future requires extraordinary faith and perseverance. It is a faith that may be tried daily, sometimes relentlessly and without much reprieve.

Author Phillip Yancey wrote, "As I visited people whose pain far exceeded my own...I was surprised by its effects."[4] He discovered that these people who were afflicted beyond what he had experienced, had actually grown closer to God and were filled with His strength. Those who stand on the outside, have difficulty understanding how a person who is suffering so greatly could possibly have a *stronger* faith in God.

The travesty is that when we should be admiring the faith of our loved one, we may very well insult their capacity to fully trust God. Stewart continued, "...the fact is that it is the world's greatest sufferers who have produced the most shining examples of unconquerable faith."[5] These people not only have their faith, but they have the faith and strength of God instilled in them to persevere through a life's stormy journey.

When we think our loved one is being weak, we tend to view that as a bad thing. However, that could be where God wants him or her so that He can be the one to sustain them. What we often fail to comprehend is that Jesus explained, "My grace is sufficient for you, for my power is made perfect in weakness." Paul continued, "Therefore I will boast all the more gladly about my weaknesses, so that Christ's power may rest on me" (2 Cor 12: 9).

When we come to Him with no strength of our own, He fills us with His might and our faith is multiplied by His grace. In fact, we cannot be filled with God until we are emptied of self (Matt 5:1). Author Peter Kreeft pointed out that "Job's suffering hollowed out a big space in him so that God and joy could fill it."[6] Spurgeon said, "You would never have known God's strength had you not been supported amid the flood waters."[7]

True, there will be many times of anguish and exhaustion, for the battle is long and constant. We should not fault our loved one when they become frustrated, depressed or even angry about their situation. God wants us to be honest with Him about our feelings. Job did that when he declared, "I will surely defend my ways to his face" (Job 13:15b) and cried out, "Therefore I will not keep silent; I will speak out in the anguish of my spirit, I will complain in the bitterness of my soul" (Job 7:11).

Job clearly showed that we can suffer, be frustrated with our condition and still have faith in God's sovereignty. Our Lord does not expect His children to always be *happy* about their affliction and neither should we. "The Bible says 'Rejoice in the Lord always' [Phil 4:4]. It doesn't say, 'Rejoice over your pain.'"[8]

When we are suffering, the Bible says, "Humble yourselves, therefore, under God's mighty hand, that he may lift you up in due time" (1 Pet 5:6). It does not say that we are to exalt ourselves; it tells us to humble ourselves *under* God's hand. It also says He will lift us up, *"in due time,"* not instantly. We must recognize that when our loved one is weakened by the journey, this is not a sign of failure.

Quite the opposite! This is where God wants us all to be - *humbled and leaning solely on Him.*

Soon we will discover that someone with a chronic condition is not someone we must fix. We will begin to see their worth right where our Lord has them today. "Instead of thinking about how far they still have to go, think about how far they have come in spite of their hurts"[9] Warren proposed.

Yes, we can continue to ask God for healing, but we must realize that God may have another plan. He may or may not choose to heal our loved one physically right here and now, therefore we must not blame our friend or family member for what God is doing.

This world is full of disease and tribulations, because it is not our home and it is not our ultimate destination. We should understand that "...life is *supposed* to be difficult! It's what enables us to grow. Remember, earth is not heaven!"[10]

"Therefore we do not lose heart. Though outwardly we are wasting away, yet inwardly we are being renewed day by day. For our light and momentary troubles are achieving for us an eternal glory that far outweighs them all. So we fix our eyes not on what is seen, but on what is unseen. For what is seen is temporary, but what is unseen is eternal" (2 Cor 4:16-18).

In all, we must realize God is in control even when we cannot see what He is doing or we do not agree with His answers. Furthermore, if we take a closer look at our loved one, their reliance upon God will inspire us and the perseverance God has given them will amaze us. Perhaps we can all learn an important lesson from our loved one living with chronic illness and pain - *how to live by faith and not by sight* (2 Cor 5:7).

Endnotes

Chapter One

[1] Lisa Lorden, "When You Need A Friend," Self published, 1999. www.anapsid.org/cnd/coping/needfriend.html (accessed March 23, 2004). Body.

[2] Pauline Boss, "Ambiguous Loss from Chronic Physical Illness: Clinical Intervention with Couples, Individuals, and Families," *Journal of Clinical Psychology-In Session, Volume 58* (November 2002): 1353.

[3] Lisa Copen, "When the Illness is Invisible," *...And He Will Give You Rest Newsletter,* Volume II, Issue 3 (1998): www.restministries.org/art-invisible.htm (accessed March 23, 2004). Body.

[4] Boss, 1352.

[5] Douglas Groothuis, "Seeing Invisible Disabilities," *MOODY,* Volume 102, No. 1 (September/October 2001): 41.

[6] Boss, 1353.

[7] F. Marcus Brown, III, "Inside Every Chronic Patient Is an Acute Patient Wondering What Happened," *Journal of Clinical Psychology-In Session, Volume 58* (November 2002): 1444.

[8] Jackson P. Rainer, "Bent but Not Broken: An Introduction to the Issue on Chronic Illness," *Journal of Clinical Psychology-In Session, Volume 58* (November 2002): 1348.

[9] Jeffrey Boyd, *But You LOOK Good!* (IDA, 2003), xiii.

Chapter Two

[1] Cathy, The Invisible Disabilities Advocate Support Board, 2001. www.InvisibleDisabilities.com (accessed 2001).

Chapter Three

[1] Copen, "When the Illness is Invisible," Introduction.

[2] Charlene, comment appeared on The Invisible Disabilities Advocate Support Board, 2000. www.InvisibleDisabilities.com (accessed 2000).

[3] Copen, "When the Illness is Invisible," Body.

[4] Copen, "When the Illness is Invisible," Body.

[5] Debbie, The Invisible Disabilities Advocate Guestbook, 2000. www.InvisibleDisabilities.com (accessed 2000).

[6] Bek Oberin, "An Open Letter to those without CFS," Self published, 2003. www.tertius.net.au/foothold/openletter.html (accessed March 23, 2004). Body.

[7] Pat, The Invisible Disabilities Advocate Survey, 1999. www.InvisibleDisabilities.com (received 1999).

[8] Lorden, "When You Need A Friend," Introduction.

[9] Copen, "When the Illness is Invisible," Introduction.

Chapter Four

[1] Linda, The Invisible Disabilities Advocate Survey, 1999. www.InvisibleDisabilities.com (received 1999).

[2] Julie, The Invisible Disabilities Advocate Guestbook, 2000. www.InvisibleDisabilities.com (received 2000).

Chapter Five

[1] Rick Warren, *The Purpose Driven Life* (Grand Rapids, Michigan: Zondervan, 2003), 199.

[2] Kathleen Lewis, "When You Accept the Illness," *...And He Will Give You Rest Newsletter*, Volume I, Issue 4 (1997): www.restministries.org/articles/art-acceptillness.htm (accessed March 23, 2004). Introduction.

[3] Lorden, "When You Need A Friend," Introduction.

[4] Oberin, "An Open Letter to those without CFS," Body.

[5] Oberin, "An Open Letter to those without CFS," Body.

[6] Oberin, "An Open Letter to those without CFS," Body.

[7] Lisa Copen, "When a Friend Has a Chronic Illness," brochure by Rest Ministries, Inc. 2001. www.restministries.org/art-whattosay.htm (accessed March 23, 2004). Body.

[8] Lewis, "When You Accept the Illness," Body.

[9] Max Lucado. "We're Not Home Yet." *A Garden in My Prison.* Audiocassette. San Antonio, Texas: UpWords, 2000.

[10] Warren, 197.

[11] Laurie Thompson, "Broken But Don't Need Fixin'," *...And He Will Give You Rest Newsletter*, Volume 5, Issue 2 (2001): www.restministries.org/articles/art-brokenbutdont.htm (accessed March 23, 2004). Conclusion.

Chapter Six

[1] Joan S. Livingston, "Perspectives on Friendship," *The Syndrome Sentinel,* 2001. www.cssa-inc.org/eNL/12-01/enewsletter.htm (accessed March 23, 2004). Body.

[2] Rainer, 1347.

[3] Brown, 1443.

4 Rainer, 1348.

5 Warren, 173.

6 Charles Spurgeon, *Morning and Evening,* (New Kensington, PA: Whitaker House, 1997), 636.

7 Warren, 194.

8 Boss, 1353.

9 Paul Borthwick, "When Pain is Your Prison," *Discipleship Journal,* Issue 139 (January/February 2004): 34.

10 Sue Klaus, "How to Kill a Sick Friend," Self published, 1996. wwcoco.com/cfids/suekkill.html (accessed March 23, 2004). Body.

Chapter Seven

1 Copen, "When a Friend Has a Chronic Illness," Body.

Chapter Eight

1 Lisa, comment appeared on The Invisible Disabilities Advocate Guestbook, 2000. www.InvisibleDisabilities.com (accessed 2000).

2 Lisa Lorden, "Some Friendly Advice," Self published, 1998. http://fmaware.org/patient/family/friendadvice.htm (accessed March 23, 2004). Body.

3 Copen, "When the Illness is Invisible," Body.

4 Boss, 1354.

5 Lisa Lorden, "Living with a Loved One with Chronic Illness: An Interview with Gregg Piburn," Self published, 2000. http://fmaware.org/patient/family/piburn.htm (accessed March 23, 2004). Body.

6 Boss, 1358.

7 Susan Dion, "Rethinking Usefulness," *The National Link,* (Winter 1995): 1-3.

8 Boss, 1351.

Chapter Nine

1 Spurgeon, 702.

2 Spurgeon, 636.

3 Warren, 194.

Barry Bridges, "Lord Kitchener and the Morant/Handcock Executions", *Journal of the Australian Historical Society* 73 (June 1987): 37.

[4] Bob Buchanan, "Hallowed Be Your Name," *The Disciple's Prayer Series*. Sermon (February 22, 2004).

Chapter Ten

[1] Oberin, "An Open Letter to those without CFS," Body.

[2] Warren, 141.

[3] Boss, 1360.

[4] Copen, "When a Friend Has a Chronic Illness," Body.

[5] Boss, 1352.

[6] Copen, "When a Friend Has a Chronic Illness," Body.

[7] Boss, 1354.

[8] Boss, 1358.

[9] Boss, 1359.

Chapter Eleven

[1] Lorden, "When You Need A Friend," Introduction.

[2] Lorden, "Some Friendly Advice," Introduction.

[3] Lorden, "Some Friendly Advice," Introduction.

[4] Warren, 141.

[5] Lorden, "Living with a Loved One with Chronic Illness: An Interview with Gregg Piburn," Body.

[6] Warren, 291

[7] Warren, 176

Chapter Thirteen

[1] Warren, 149

[2] Livingston, "Perspectives on Friendship," Body.

[3] Warren, 126

[4] Lisa Copen, "How Do I Make People Understand?" *...And He Will Give You Rest Newsletter,* Volume 5, Issue 6 (2001): www.restministries.org/articles/art-makepeopleunderstand.htm (accessed March 23, 2004). Body.

[5] Warren, 141

Chapter Fourteen

[1] Warren, 194

[2] Warren W. Wiersbe, *Classic Sermons on Suffering* (Grand Rapids, Mich.: Kregel Publications, 1984), 92.

[3] Warren, 198.

[4] Philip Yancey, *Where Is God When It Hurts?* (Grand Rapids, Mich.: Zondervan, 1990), 255-256.

[5] Wiersbe, 92.

[6] Lee Strobel, *The Case for Faith* (Grand Rapids, Mich.: Zondervan, 2000), 50.

[7] Spurgeon, 636.

[8] Warren, 199

[9] Warren, 149

[10] Warren, 173

References

Borthwick, Paul. "When Pain is Your Prison." *Discipleship Journal,* Issue 139 (January/February 2004). Paul's website address is: www.borthwicks.org.

Boss, Pauline. "Ambiguous Loss from Chronic Physical Illness: Clinical Intervention with Couples, Individuals, and Families." *Journal of Clinical Psychology-In Session*, Volume 58 (2002): 1351-1360.

Boyd, Jeffrey. "A Tribute to an American Heroine." Foreword from the book: *But You LOOK Good: A Guide to Understanding and Encouraging People Living With Chronic Illness and Pain!* Colorado: The Invisible Disabilities Advocate, 2003. The Invisible Disabilities Advocate: www.MyIDA.org

Brown, F. Marcus III (November 2002). "Inside Every Chronic Patient is and Acute Patient Wondering What Happened." *Journal of Clinical Psychology-In Session,* Volume 58 (2002): 1443-1449.

Buchanan, Bob Buchanan. "Hallowed Be Your Name." *The Disciple's Prayer Series.* Sermon. Personal Communications (February 22, 2004).

Copen, Lisa. "How Do I Make People Understand?" *...And He Will Give You Rest Newsletter,* Volume V, Issue 6 (2001). Copen is the Founder of Rest Ministries: www.RestMinistries.org.

Copen, Lisa. *When a Friend Has a Chronic Illness.* Brochure Distributed By Rest Ministries (2001). Copen is the Founder of Rest Ministries: www.RestMinistries.org.

Copen, Lisa. "When the Illness is Invisible." *...And He Will Give You Rest Newsletter,* Volume II, Issue 3 (1998). Copen is the Founder of Rest Ministries: www.RestMinistries.org.

Dion, Susan. "Rethinking Usefulness." *The National Link*, Winter 1995. Dion is the author of *WRITE NOW: Maintaining A Creative Spirit While Homebound and Ill.*

The Invisible Disabilities Advocate Guestbook. Comments posted by visitors to the IDA Website in a public format of a guestbook (1998-2001). All published quotes were given publicly and/or permission was granted.

The Invisible Disabilities Advocate Support Board. Comments posted by visitors to the IDA Website in a public format of a message board (2001). Permission to publish granted.

The Invisible Disabilities Advocate Survey. An Informal question, "How Does Your Church Deal With Illness?" was posed to various health-related support forums, clubs and message boards on the Internet (November 1999). Permission to publish agreed to by those who responded to the survey.

Lewis, Kathleen. "When You Accept the Illness," ...And He Will Give You Rest Newsletter, Volume I, Issue 4 (1997). Article adapted from Successful Living with Chronic Illness, re-titled, *Celebrate Life*. Celebrate Life website: www.LetsCelebrateLife.com

Groothuis, Doug. "Seeing Invisible Disabilities." *MOODY*, Volume 102 (2001). Visit Dr. Groothuis' website at: www.gospelcom.net/ivpress/groothuis/

Klaus, Sue. "How to Kill a Sick Friend." Self Published (1996). *Listening to CFIDS*. www.coco.com/cfids (accessed March 23, 2004).

Livingston, Joan S. "Perspectives On Friendship." Self Published (2001). *The Syndrome Sentinel* (December, 2001). *The Chronic Syndrome Support* Association. www.cssa-inc.org (accessed March 23, 2004).

Lorden, Lisa. "Some Friendly Advice." Self Published (1998). *National Fibromyalgia Association*. http://fmaware.org/patient/family/friendadvice.htm (accessed March 23, 2004). Lorden is a writer who lives with CFIDS and FMS.

Lorden, Lisa. "When You Need A Friend." Self published (1999). *Melissa Kaplan's Chronic Neuroimmune Diseases*. www.anapsid.org/cnd/coping/needfriend.html (accessed March 23, 2004). Lorden is a writer who lives with CFIDS and FMS.

Lorden, Lisa. "Living with a Loved One with Chronic Illness: An Interview with Gregg Piburn." Self Published (2000). *National Fibromyalgia Association*. http://fmaware.org/patient/family/piburn.htm (accessed March 23, 2004). Lorden is a writer who lives with CFIDS and FMS. Gregg Piburn, is the author of *Beyond Chaos: One Man's Journey Alongside His Chronically Ill Wife*. You may contact Gregg at: gpiburn@msn.com or through his website: www.LeadersEdgeConsulting.com. You may order *Beyond Chaos* from the Arthritis Foundation: 1-800-207-8633.

Lucado, Max. "We're Not Home Yet." *A Garden in My Prison*. Sermon Series. Audiocassette. San Antonio, Texas: UpWords, 2000. Copyrighted material used with permission from UpWords 4/25/2001.

Oberin, Bek. "An Open Letter to Those Without Fibro/CFS." Self Published (2003). *Fibro/CFS Foothold*. http://tertius.net.au/foothold/openletter.html (accessed March 23, 2004). Oberin is the author of *The Fibro/CFS* Foothold Website: http://minerva.tertius.net.au/foothold. Quotes published with permission.

Rainer, Jackson P. "Bent but Not Broken: An Introduction to the Issue on Chronic Illness." *Journal of Clinical Psychology-In Session,* Volume 58 (2002): 1347-1350.

Spurgeon, Charles. *Morning & Evening*. New Kensington, PA: Whitaker House, 1997. Copyrighted material printed with permission from Whitaker House 5/31/2001.

Strobel, Lee. *The Case for Faith*. Grand Rapids Michigan: Zondervan Publishing House, 2000. Used by permission of The Zondervan Corporation.

Thompson, Laurie. "Broken but Don't Need Fixin'." *...And He Will Give You Rest Newsletter,* Volume 5, Issue 2 (2001).

Warren, Rick. *The Purpose Driven Life*. Grand Rapids, Michigan: Zondervan, 2002. Used by permission of The Zondervan Corporation.

Wiersbe, Warren. *Classic Sermons on Suffering*. Grand Rapids, Michigan: Kregel Publications, 1984.

Yancey, Philip. *Where is God When it Hurts?* Grand Rapids, Michigan: Zondervan, 1990. Used by permission of The Zondervan Corporation.

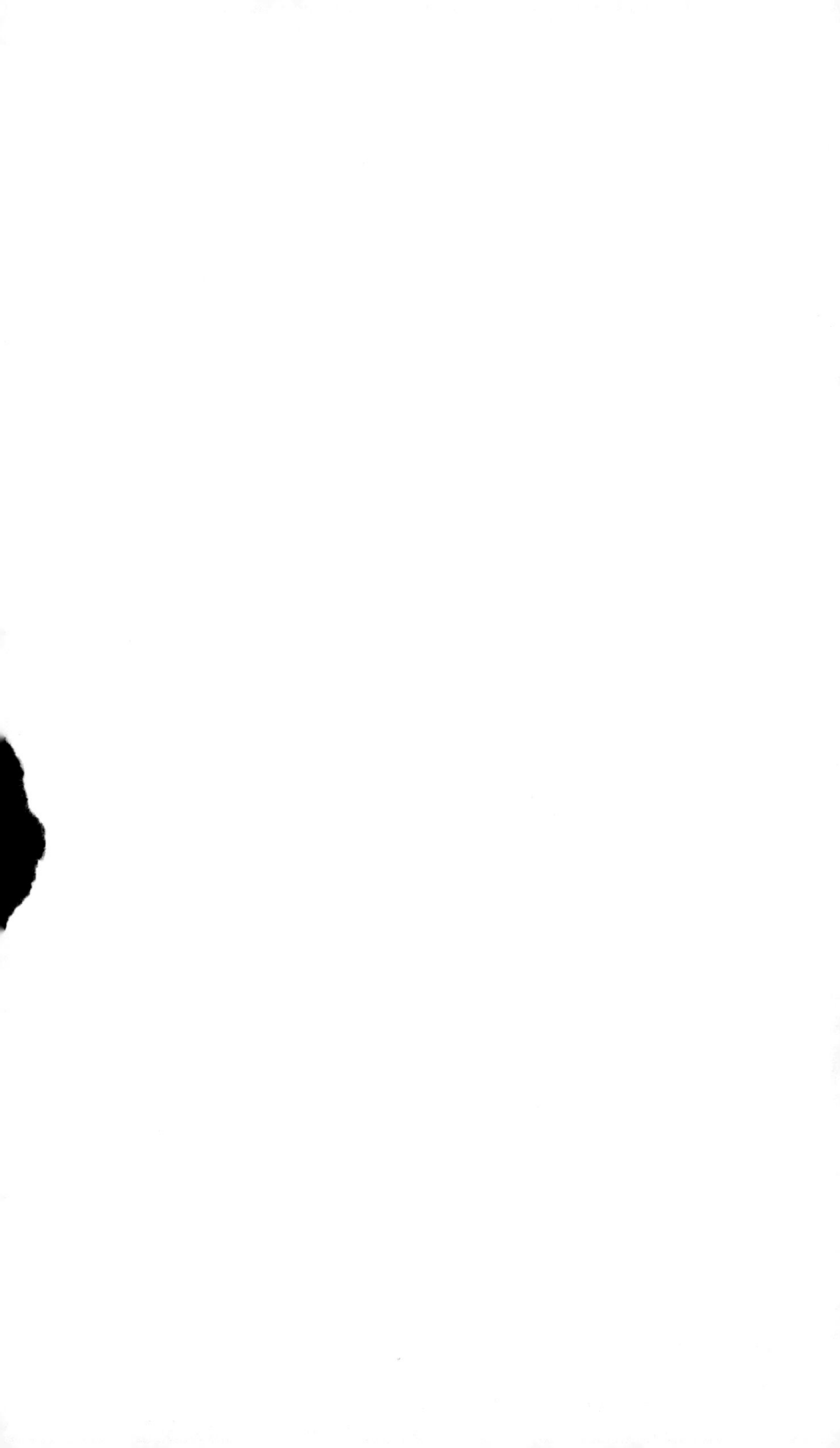

www.ingramcontent.com/pod-product-compliance
Lightning Source LLC
Chambersburg PA
CBHW060945040426
42445CB00011B/1006